**COGNITIVE-BEHAVIORAL
CONJOINT THERAPY
FOR PTSD**

# Also from Candice M. Monson

For more information, visit the authors' website: *www.coupletherapyforptsd.com*

*Couple-Based Interventions for Military and Veteran Families:*
*A Practitioner's Guide*
EDITED BY DOUGLAS K. SNYDER AND CANDICE M. MONSON

# Cognitive-Behavioral Conjoint Therapy for PTSD

**Harnessing the Healing Power of Relationships**

Candice M. Monson
Steffany J. Fredman

**THE GUILFORD PRESS**
New York   London

© 2012 The Guilford Press
A Division of Guilford Publications, Inc.
370 Seventh Avenue, Suite 1200, New York, NY 10001
www.guilford.com

All rights reserved

Except as noted, no part of this book may be reproduced, translated, stored in a retrieval system, or transmitted, in any form or by any means, electronic, mechanical, photocopying, microfilming, recording, or otherwise, without written permission from the publisher.

Printed in the United States of America

This book is printed on acid-free paper.

Last digit is print number:  9  8  7  6

---

LIMITED PHOTOCOPY LICENSE

These materials are intended for use only by qualified mental health professionals.

The publisher grants to individual purchasers of this book nonassignable permission to reproduce all materials for which photocopying permission is specifically granted in a footnote. This license is limited to you, the individual purchaser, for personal use or use with individual clients. This license does not grant the right to reproduce these materials for resale, redistribution, electronic display, or any other purposes (including but not limited to books, pamphlets, articles, video- or audiotapes, blogs, file-sharing sites, Internet or intranet sites, and handouts or slides for lectures, workshops, or webinars, whether or not a fee is charged). Permission to reproduce these materials for these and any other purposes must be obtained in writing from the Permissions Department of Guilford Publications.

---

The authors have checked with sources believed to be reliable in their efforts to provide information that is complete and generally in accord with the standards of practice that are accepted at the time of publication. However, in view of the possibility of human error or changes in behavioral, mental health, or medical sciences, neither the authors, nor the editor and publisher, nor any other party who has been involved in the preparation or publication of this work warrants that the information contained herein is in every respect accurate or complete, and they are not responsible for any errors or omissions or the results obtained from the use of such information. Readers are encouraged to confirm the information contained in this book with other sources.

**Library of Congress Cataloging-in-Publication Data**

Monson, Candice M.
  Cognitive-behavioral conjoint therapy for PTSD : harnessing the healing power of relationships / Candice M. Monson, Steffany J. Fredman.
    p. cm.
  Includes bibliographical references and index.
  ISBN 978-1-4625-0553-1 (pbk. : alk. paper)
   1. Post-traumatic stress disorder—Treatment.   2. Cognitive therapy.   3. Couples therapy.
 4. Post-traumatic stress disorder—Patients—Family relationships.   I. Fredman, Steffany J.   II. Title.
  RC552.P67M66 2012
  616.85′21—dc23

2012013188

# About the Authors

**Candice M. Monson, PhD,** is Professor of Psychology and Director of Clinical Training at Toronto Metropolitan University. She is also an Affiliate of the Women's Health Sciences Division of the U.S. Department of Veterans Affairs National Center for Posttraumatic Stress Disorder, where she previously served as Deputy Director. Dr. Monson is one of the foremost experts on intimate relationships and traumatic stress and the use of conjoint therapy to treat posttraumatic stress disorder (PTSD). She has published extensively on the development, evaluation, and dissemination of PTSD treatments more generally as well as gender differences in violence perpetration and victimization. She has been funded by the U.S. Department of Veteran Affairs, the National Institute of Mental Health, the Centers for Disease Control and Prevention, the U.S. Department of Defense, and the Canadian Institutes of Health for her research on interpersonal factors in traumatization and couple-based interventions for PTSD. Dr. Monson is coauthor of *Cognitive Processing Therapy: Veteran/Military Version*, coeditor of *Couple-Based Interventions for Military and Veteran Families*, and the codeveloper of cognitive-behavioral conjoint therapy for PTSD.

**Steffany J. Fredman, PhD,** is Assistant Professor of Human Development and Family Studies at the Pennsylvania State University. Dr. Fredman is a recipient of the Martin S. Wallach Award for Outstanding Doctoral Candidate in Clinical Psychology from the University of North Carolina at Chapel Hill. Her clinical and research interests focus on the interpersonal context of individual psychopathology with an emphasis on PTSD, and her work has been funded by the National Institute of Mental Health. Dr. Fredman is the codeveloper of cognitive-behavioral conjoint therapy for PTSD and is currently adapting this treatment model for telehealth delivery as a way to increase access to care for traumatized individuals and their significant others.

# Preface

We began developing this conjoint therapy for posttraumatic stress disorder (PTSD) at the end of the 1990s. Its development grew out of our observation that too little attention had been paid to the inherently interpersonal nature of traumatization and the strong relational influences and ramifications of traumatic-stress-related problems when they manifest. At present, most of the treatments disseminated for PTSD and its common comorbidities are individually focused. Although efficacious for improving PTSD and its common comorbid mental health symptoms, these treatments show minimal effects on intimate relationships, broader family relations, friendships, and general interpersonal functioning. Yet, one's relationships are often the catalyst to get help, important sources of support or stress, and the very parts of people's lives that they most want to change. This therapy seeks to harness the potential healing power of clients' interactions with significant others to improve posttraumatic reactions and experiences within those relationships.

We would be remiss if we did not credit several innovative clinical researchers and practitioners for their intellectual influence on the development of our treatment and this book. We are grateful to the couple/family colleagues who came before us and paved the road for the use of conjoint and family interventions for a variety of individual problems, including PTSD (e.g., Donald Baucom, Shirley Glynn, David Miklowitz, Timothy O'Farrell, Neil Jacobson, K. Daniel O'Leary, and Douglas Snyder). Patricia Resick and Kathleen Chard have been extremely influential and generous in their contributions to our "thinking about" PTSD and how to develop a cognitive therapy for PTSD that can be effectively delivered in a dyadic format. Cognitive processing therapy (Resick, Monson, & Chard, 2007) is integral to the content found in the final stage of our treatment. We have also drawn on Steven Hayes and Kelly Wilson's innovative work on the phenomenon of experiential avoidance. We have used this framework to develop treatment interventions that allow traumatized individuals and their loved ones to develop tolerance for the affective states associated with their traumas, within a conjoint context.

We also appreciate the instrumental and emotional support of our colleagues at the VA National Center for Posttraumatic Stress Disorder, Executive and Women's Health Sciences Divisions, in this endeavor. Paula Schnurr is to be credited for being the first to support the notion of our developing this treatment and for her unwavering support of it since. She was integral to a more nuanced and rich conceptualization of the theory that supports the therapy.

Also thank you to Susan Stevens and Karen Guthrie for their early contributions to the therapy and its provision and to Carrie Adair and Jennifer Belus for their tireless formatting and reformatting of the protocol. In addition, we are deeply grateful to our own spouses, children, and other family members for supporting us along this journey and, through their love, devotion, and "big-picture thinking," for reminding us on a daily basis that a caring relationship helps to sustain and heal despite the challenges we may encounter.

Finally, we owe much to the traumatized individuals and their loved ones who have allowed us into their lives to learn from them and to share the hope of better lives and relationships.

# Contents

List of Handouts     xi

## PART I. BACKGROUND AND OVERVIEW OF CBCT FOR PTSD

CHAPTER 1. An Introduction to Cognitive-Behavioral Conjoint Therapy for PTSD     3

CHAPTER 2. Initial Assessment, Case Conceptualization, and Working with Complex Cases     26

## PART II. CBCT FOR PTSD TREATMENT MANUAL

### PHASE 1. RATIONALE FOR TREATMENT AND EDUCATION ABOUT PTSD AND RELATIONSHIPS

SESSION 1. Introduction to Treatment     53

SESSION 2. Safety Building     73

### PHASE 2. SATISFACTION ENHANCEMENT AND UNDERMINING AVOIDANCE

SESSION 3. Listening and Approaching     93

SESSION 4. Sharing Thoughts and Feelings: Emphasis on *Feelings*     105

SESSION 5. Sharing Thoughts and Feelings: Emphasis on *Thoughts*     118

SESSION 6. Getting U.N.S.T.U.C.K.     126

SESSION 7. Problem Solving to Shrink PTSD     138

### PHASE 3. MAKING MEANING OF THE TRAUMA(S) AND END OF THERAPY

SESSION 8. Acceptance     151

SESSION 9. Blame     165

| SESSION 10. | Trust | 179 |
|---|---|---|
| SESSION 11. | Control | 189 |
| SESSION 12. | Emotional Closeness | 197 |
| SESSION 13. | Physical Closeness | 205 |
| SESSION 14. | Posttraumatic Growth | 213 |
| SESSION 15. | Review and Reinforcement of Treatment Gains | 224 |

| References | 229 |
|---|---|
| Index | 235 |

# List of Handouts

| HANDOUT 1.1 | Cognitive-Behavioral Conjoint Therapy for PTSD: Session Overview | 63 |
| HANDOUT 1.2 | Cycle of PTSD Symptoms and Recovery from Trauma | 64 |
| HANDOUT 1.3 | Treatment Contract | 65 |
| HANDOUT 1.4 | Trauma and Relationships | 67 |
| HANDOUT 1.5 | Trauma Impact Questions–I | 70 |
| HANDOUT 1.6 | Out-of-Session Assignments: Session 1. Introduction to Treatment | 72 |
| HANDOUT 2.1 | Learning about Anger | 87 |
| HANDOUT 2.2 | Steps to an Effective Time-Out | 88 |
| HANDOUT 2.3 | Out-of-Session Assignments: Session 2. Safety Building | 89 |
| HANDOUT 3.1 | PTSD and Avoidance | 102 |
| HANDOUT 3.2 | Avoidance List | 103 |
| HANDOUT 3.3 | Out-of-Session Assignments: Session 3. Listening and Approaching | 104 |
| HANDOUT 4.1 | Communication Channels | 114 |
| HANDOUT 4.2 | Identifying Feelings | 115 |
| HANDOUT 4.3 | PROUD to Shrink PTSD: Getting the Most Out of Your Approach Tasks | 116 |

| | | |
|---|---|---|
| **HANDOUT 4.4** | Out-of-Session Assignments: Session 4. Sharing Thoughts and Feelings: Emphasis on *Feelings* | 117 |
| **HANDOUT 5.1** | Sharing Thoughts and Feelings to Shrink PTSD | 123 |
| **HANDOUT 5.2** | Catch Your Partner's Thoughts and Feelings | 124 |
| **HANDOUT 5.3** | Out-of-Session Assignments: Session 5. Sharing Thoughts and Feelings: Emphasis on *Thoughts* | 125 |
| **HANDOUT 6.1** | Getting U.N.S.T.U.C.K. | 134 |
| **HANDOUT 6.2** | The Big Picture | 135 |
| **HANDOUT 6.3** | Catch Your Partner's Thoughts and Feelings | 136 |
| **HANDOUT 6.4** | Out-of-Session Assignments: Session 6. Getting U.N.S.T.U.C.K. | 137 |
| **HANDOUT 7.1** | Problem-Solving/Decision-Making Guidelines | 146 |
| **HANDOUT 7.2** | The Big Picture | 147 |
| **HANDOUT 7.3** | Out-of-Session Assignments: Session 7. Problem Solving to Shrink PTSD | 148 |
| **HANDOUT 8.1** | Stuck Point List | 161 |
| **HANDOUT 8.2** | Barriers to Acceptance | 162 |
| **HANDOUT 8.3** | The Big Picture | 163 |
| **HANDOUT 8.4** | Out-of-Session Assignments: Session 8. Getting U.N.S.T.U.C.K. to Promote Acceptance | 164 |
| **HANDOUT 9.1** | Getting U.N.S.T.U.C.K. Regarding Blame | 176 |
| **HANDOUT 9.2** | The Big Picture | 177 |
| **HANDOUT 9.3** | Out-of-Session Assignments: Session 9. Getting U.N.S.T.U.C.K. Regarding Blame | 178 |
| **HANDOUT 10.1** | Getting U.N.S.T.U.C.K. Regarding Trust | 185 |
| **HANDOUT 10.2** | The Big Picture | 187 |
| **HANDOUT 10.3** | Out-of-Session Assignments: Session 10. Getting U.N.S.T.U.C.K. Regarding Trust | 188 |
| **HANDOUT 11.1** | Getting U.N.S.T.U.C.K. Regarding Control | 194 |

| **HANDOUT 11.2** | The Big Picture | 195 |
| --- | --- | --- |
| **HANDOUT 11.3** | Out-of-Session Assignments: Session 11. Getting U.N.S.T.U.C.K. Regarding Control | 196 |
| **HANDOUT 12.1** | Getting U.N.S.T.U.C.K. Regarding Emotional Closeness | 202 |
| **HANDOUT 12.2** | The Big Picture | 203 |
| **HANDOUT 12.3** | Out-of-Session Assignments: Session 12. Getting U.N.S.T.U.C.K. Regarding Emotional Closeness | 204 |
| **HANDOUT 13.1** | Getting U.N.S.T.U.C.K. Regarding Physical Closeness | 210 |
| **HANDOUT 13.2** | The Big Picture | 211 |
| **HANDOUT 13.3** | Out-of-Session Assignments: Session 13. Getting U.N.S.T.U.C.K. Regarding Physical Closeness | 212 |
| **HANDOUT 14.1** | Getting U.N.S.T.U.C.K. Regarding Posttraumatic Growth | 218 |
| **HANDOUT 14.2** | The Big Picture | 219 |
| **HANDOUT 14.3** | Trauma Impact Questions–II | 220 |
| **HANDOUT 14.4** | What Have We Learned? | 222 |
| **HANDOUT 14.5** | Out-of-Session Assignments: Session 14. Getting U.N.S.T.U.C.K. Regarding Posttraumatic Growth | 223 |

# COGNITIVE-BEHAVIORAL CONJOINT THERAPY FOR PTSD

# PART I

# BACKGROUND AND OVERVIEW OF CBCT FOR PTSD

# CHAPTER 1

# An Introduction to Cognitive-Behavioral Conjoint Therapy for PTSD

Approximately 75% of North Americans will be exposed to a traumatic event at some point in their lifetime that could lead to posttraumatic stress disorder (PTSD; Kessler, Sonnega, Bromet, Hughes, & Nelson, 1995). Of these individuals, about 8% will be diagnosed with PTSD in their lifetime, and many more will have symptoms of the disorder. Symptoms of PTSD include reexperiencing (i.e., reliving the event through intrusive memories, nightmares, flashbacks, distress at reminders), avoidance (i.e., active avoidance of reminders in the environment), emotional numbing (i.e., difficulty feeling a range of positive and negative emotions), and hyperarousal (i.e., sleep disturbances, anger/irritability, exaggerated startle, hypervigilance, concentration difficulties). Left untreated, these symptoms most often have a chronic and pernicious course associated with substantial individual and societal costs (Greenberg et al., 1999; Kessler, 2000).

Most theories, empirical research, and treatments to date have focused on the intrapersonal facets of PTSD. For example, individual psychophysiology, brain structure and functioning, personality traits, and cognitive styles are frequent topics of study. Current treatments identified in guidelines for the effective treatment of PTSD are delivered individually (Foa, Keane, & Friedman, 2009; Institute of Medicine, 2007; Veterans Health Administration, U.S. Department of Defense, 2004). With this text, we offer a new approach to the treatment of PTSD—cognitive-behavioral conjoint therapy (CBCT) for PTSD—that capitalizes on our growing recognition of the interpersonal nature and consequences of trauma and the potential power of intimate relationships to ameliorate PTSD. This is especially timely, given the rising rates of violence, the ongoing threat and realities of man-made and natural disasters, and the continued military involvement around the world that can have broad and devastating effects on individuals and their loved ones (Centers for Disease Control and Prevention, National Center for Injury Prevention and Control, 2011; Norris, Friedman, & Watson, 2002; Norris, Friedman, Watson, Byrne, et al., 2002; North, Kawasaki, Spitznagel, & Hong, 2004).

CBCT for PTSD is a time-limited, manualized, disorder-specific conjoint therapy with the simultaneous goals of improving PTSD and enhancing intimate relationship functioning. We have evidence that this therapy also improves co-occurring conditions and the mental health and well-being of close others who participate in the therapy with a loved one with posttraumatic stress problems (see Chapter 2 for a review). CBCT for PTSD is designed to be a stand-alone treatment for PTSD; that is, it is not intended to be delivered as an adjunctive therapy to individual PTSD treatment. It is also not a conjoint therapy to be provided after a course of individual PTSD therapy unless individual PTSD treatment did not result in intended improvements.

CBCT for PTSD is designed for couples with a range of relationship satisfaction levels, and not only for distressed couples. In other words, couples do not need to have clinical levels of relationship distress to profit from the treatment. In the majority of couples presenting for treatment, at least some relationship distress will be the norm, and they may have already discussed the possibility of dissolving the relationship or may be ambivalent about remaining together. In these cases, the benefit of a conjoint treatment to address PTSD is readily apparent. Nonetheless, it is our experience that even highly satisfied couples in which at least one partner has PTSD are in need of a conjoint treatment format, because the structure and the function of their relationship maintain the individual mental health problems. Family relationship systems that have rigid rules and expectations about how partners will function in the relationship can be less receptive to individual change in therapy. Referred to by some as *symptom–system fit* (Baucom, Stanton, & Epstein, 2003; Rohrbaugh, Shoham, Spungen, & Steinglass, 1985), individual changes may be resisted by the couple or family system. For example, a spouse may discourage her partner with PTSD from facing trauma reminders, and thereby improving, because she is gratified by the notion of being the caregiver of an "ill" spouse. Conjoint treatments such as CBCT for PTSD are able to address the relational system that may contribute to or maintain individual psychopathology.

The clients whom we and others have treated with CBCT for PTSD have suffered a range of traumatic events, from childhood and adult sexual and physical assault to military combat and peacekeeping missions to the witnessing of genocide to the loss of loved ones by sudden death as well as a combination of events. We have used CBCT for PTSD with many dyads in which both individuals have experienced trauma and in which both individuals were diagnosed with PTSD. We also have conducted the therapy with different types of dyads: heterosexual and gay couples, cohabitating and noncohabitating couples, and even nonromantic dyads, such as siblings and close friends. We have treated couples who have dated for only months to couples who have been married more than 25 years. At the outset, we titled the therapy a "conjoint" versus "couple" therapy because we envisioned its application to a range of traumatized individuals and the loved ones whom they considered closest to them. In Chapter 2 we discuss implementation of the protocol with these different types of dyads and the issues that they can bring, which are a point of focus for the therapy.

Although originally developed and tested as a treatment for PTSD, we have since found this therapy to lead to improvements in a range of mental health problems that arise after traumatization, including depression, substance use, guilt, anger, dissociation, and other anxiety symptoms (panic, general anxiety). The range of traumatic stress problems also needs to be conceptualized and addressed in treatment to optimize outcomes. For example, if there is comorbid substance abuse or dissociation, these symptoms need to be assessed, monitored, and addressed throughout the therapy. We discuss conceptualization of these problems within the therapy and comment on their intervention throughout the protocol.

It is important to note that CBCT for PTSD is a trauma-focused treatment, but it does not include imaginal exposure-based interventions (i.e., repeatedly imagining the traumatic event until anxiety surrounding the memory subsides). When discussing the trauma memory in the final phase of treatment, couples are discouraged from discussing nitty-gritty or explicit renditions of traumatic events. In keeping with a cognitive approach to processing the trauma, we and others have found that discussing the traumas as if from a "10,000-foot view" provides enough detail to facilitate shifts in the ways patients and their significant others think about the event and its consequences (Resick, Monson, & Chard, 2008). In this way, clients are able to process the memory by properly contextualizing the event and correcting any misappraisals about it—the goal of CBCT for PTSD. Patients are encouraged to engage in traditionally described *in vivo* exposure exercises (e.g., Foa, Hembree, & Rothbaum, 2007), which we describe as approach assignments that are either completed as a couple or conceptualized within an interpersonal framework (e.g., sometimes partners serve as safety signals, and the approach assignments involve removing the partner from certain places and situations). These assignments are designed to create new learning about current situations, places, people, and feelings that are reminiscent of the traumatic event but are, in fact, safe.

## Benefits of Conjoint Therapy for PTSD

Given the available choices for the treatment of traumatic stress-related problems, why have clinicians and clients alike chosen to pursue CBCT for PTSD? Why might you deliver this therapy to your clients?

There are a number of benefits of conjoint therapy for PTSD, all derived from its focus on the importance of interpersonal factors in PTSD, based on evidence regarding intimate relationships and individual PTSD treatment, the role of loved ones in PTSD treatment engagement and retention, and the efficacy of CBCT for PTSD (see Chapter 2).

### *The Importance of Interpersonal Factors in PTSD*

The majority of traumatic experiences that lead to PTSD occur at the hands of others. In fact, the two types of traumatic events most likely to lead to PTSD are man-made: rape and combat exposure (Kessler et al., 1995). Other human-induced traumatic experiences can also precipitate PTSD, including, for example, physical aggression, motor vehicle accidents, and witnessing violence (e.g., assault, witnessing murder). By their nature, these experiences can lead to a range of interpersonal disruptions. In a related vein, Freyd and colleagues (e.g., Freyd, 1996) have written extensively about the specific sequelae of "betrayal traumas," or traumas that involve betrayal by persons or institutions that one depends on for survival. This class of traumas has been shown to be particularly deleterious to individual and interpersonal functioning (e.g., Birrell & Freyd, 2006).

When a trauma is not man-made but results from a natural or technological disaster, it is simultaneously experienced with others, and the circumstances that follow in the wake of trauma are interpersonally situated. Hurricane Katrina is a salient example. Individuals and families sought refuge together as the levees broke and water surged, and they worked together (or not) to survive until the water receded. Many people expressed dismay and betrayal at the response of the U.S. federal and state agencies to provide safe water, food, and temporary housing for people affected by the storm, believing that this disaster could have been prevented outright or at least mitigated once it occurred. Because these and other traumatic experiences occur in an interpersonal context, it is important to take into account interpersonally contextualized behaviors, emotions, and beliefs linked to traumatization in order to treat the sequelae of traumatic experiences most effectively.

Consistent with the inherently interpersonal nature of traumatization, posttrauma social support has consistently emerged as one of the most potent factors associated with PTSD and other trauma-related mental health disorders. By now, there have been several meta-analyses of factors associated with PTSD after exposure to traumatic events. Brewin, Andrews, and Valentine (2000) found that the pretrauma factors of female sex, social, educational, intellectual disadvantage, and psychiatric history were associated with PTSD. However, trauma intensity and posttrauma factors had larger effects on the risk for later PTSD than did pretrauma variables. Trauma severity, lack of social support, and additional life stress were especially strongly associated with PTSD, with lack of social support being the greatest.

Ozer, Best, Lipsey, and Weiss (2003), in their meta-analysis of factors associated with PTSD in adults, investigated seven predictors: (1) prior trauma, (2) prior psychological problems, (3) family history of psychopathology, (4) perceived life threat during the trauma, (5) posttrauma social support, (6) peritraumatic emotional responses, and (7) peritraumatic dissociation. They found that all of the variables were significantly associated with PTSD: Peritraumatic dissociation and social support had the strongest associations and, consistent with Brewin and colleagues (2000), family history, prior trauma, and prior adjustment had the weakest. Interestingly, Ozer et al. also found that the association between poor social support and PTSD symptomatology was *stronger* with greater lapse of time after traumatization, suggesting that the buffering effects of social support may be cumulative over time or that the symptoms of chronic PTSD may, in fact, erode social support.

The notion that symptoms of PTSD and its comorbidities may erode social support has been validated by several studies of war veterans and disaster victims. For example, cross-sectional studies of Vietnam War (Keane, Scott, Chavoya, Lamparski, & Fairbank, 1985; King, King, Fairbank, Keane, & Adams, 1998) and Persian Gulf War (King, Taft, King, Hammond, & Stone, 2006) veterans have shown that chronic PTSD symptoms erode social support more than vice versa. Another study examined the association between social support and PTSD over time in the more acute phases of disaster recovery (Kaniasty & Norris, 2008). The researchers interviewed survivors of a flood that devastated a number of communities in Mexico in 1999. They found that familial social support predicted PTSD symptoms between 6 and 12 months posttrauma but that this was reversed between 18 and 24 months posttrauma. Between 12 and 18 months posttrauma, a bidirectional association between social support and PTSD symptoms emerged. Regardless of directionality, there is a strong association between poor social support and PTSD symptoms, possibly more so than any other variable.

## *The Role of Family Functioning in Individual PTSD Treatment and Vice Versa*

Conventional clinical wisdom holds that individual PTSD treatment will result in cascading improvements in interpersonal functioning. With this line of thinking, treatment planning often involves providing couple/family therapy after the individual PTSD treatment if it is needed.

Empirical data, however, have not supported the notion that individual PTSD treatment will necessarily ameliorate couple/family problems. Monson and colleagues' (2006) trial of individual cognitive processing therapy for military-related PTSD did not reveal significant improvements in many areas of psychosocial functioning, including close relationship functioning, as a result of treatment. Thus, in order for interpersonal relationships to improve, it does not seem sufficient to focus solely on treating PTSD symptoms.

If individual PTSD treatment does not generally improve relationship functioning, does relationship functioning influence individual PTSD treatment? The answer seems to be "yes." Two studies have examined the role of couple or family functioning in individual PTSD treatment outcomes. In their study of individual imaginal exposure and cognitive therapy for PTSD, Tarrier, Sommerfield, and Pilgram (1999) found that patients whose relatives displayed high levels of criticism and/or hostility (i.e., high expressed emotion) exhibited significantly less improvement in PTSD symptoms, depressive symptoms, and general anxiety following treatment than did those with relatives who expressed low levels of these behaviors.

Similarly, Monson, Rodriguez, and Warner (2005) studied the role of interpersonal relationship variables in two forms of group CBT for veterans with PTSD: trauma focused (i.e., exposure to trauma memories and cognitive restructuring of trauma-related beliefs) and skills focused (i.e., symptom management skills without focus on traumatic memories and reminders). Although there were no differences in the PTSD outcomes for the two forms of treatment, pretreatment intimate relationship functioning was more strongly associated with treatment outcomes in the trauma- versus skills-focused therapy. In the trauma-focused group, there was a stronger association between pretreatment intimate relationship functioning and intimate violence perpetration outcomes. Greater intimate relationship adjustment at pretreatment was associated with lower levels of intimate violence perpetration at follow-up for veterans who received trauma-focused versus skills-focused treatment. These studies suggest that there are benefits to enhancing the interpersonal milieu of those who are endeavoring PTSD treatment, particularly trauma-focused treatment.

## *Benefits for Treatment Engagement and Retention*

Despite years of public health campaigns to decrease the stigma surrounding mental health problems, there is still significant evidence of its effects in preventing people from seeking sorely needed services. Nowhere is this more apparent than among active-duty service members and veterans of the Iraq and Afghanistan Wars. Several academic articles have been written about the need to overcome the stigma among service members and veterans about seeking mental health services (Dickstein, Vogt, Handa, & Litz, 2010; Hoge, Castro, & Messer, 2004). Military policies have even been revised to help overcome this stigma and protect service members' careers when they seek mental health services. Yet it is our experience that, for a variety of reasons, military and community members alike are loathe to admit to individual problems and to seek treatment.

Individuals presenting for our therapy have appreciated the option of being able to say they are seeking couple or family therapy rather than individual therapy for a mental health disorder. Patients have expressed that it has been less stigmatizing for them to engage in this mode of therapy. One police officer who completed the treatment with his wife commented, "If this would have been individual counseling, I would have never gotten help. I would have never shown up." From the time people seek assessment and treatment, we present traumatic stress-related problems as existing in an interpersonal context, and not within either of them, in order to overcome stigma, increase buy-in, and decrease the mutual blame that often exists in these dyads. We believe couple/family therapies are often overlooked as an important conduit to treatment for many people who are reluctant to seek services for individually defined problems.

When individuals seek treatment for PTSD, a relative minority present because of the symptoms of PTSD per se. In most cases, individuals with mental health problems, including PTSD, depression, and substance use disorders, ultimately seek treatment because of psychosocial impairments associated with these disorders: for example, marital dysfunction leading to threats of divorce, struggles in their interaction with their children, employment-related trouble, or legal problems. It is often these functional impairments that get people to treatment and may, in the longer term, keep them in treatment. We believe that meeting clients "where it hurts" in their daily life is more likely to lead to treatment engagement and motivation to improve the psychopathology driving those impairments. Interpersonal problems are a significant source of "where it hurts" for clients with trauma-related symptoms and their loved ones.

Decades of research have validated the association between traumatic stress-related problems and intimate relationship functioning. For example, these studies indicate that those diagnosed with PTSD are three to six times more likely to divorce than those without PTSD (Davidson, Hughes, Blazer, & George, 1991; Kessler, Walters, & Forthofer, 1998). An epidemiological study of nearly 5,000 spouses in Ontario, Canada, investigated the association between nine mental health diagnoses and marital distress (Whisman, Sheldon, & Goering, 2000). The authors found that clinical levels of marital distress were 3.8 times more likely among couples with a partner diagnosed with PTSD, a rate second only to that for a diagnosis of dysthmia (5.7 times). A number of cross-sectional studies with clinical samples reveal that the severity of PTSD symptoms is associated with the number and severity of relationship problems, level of self-disclosure and expressiveness between partners, and degree of anxiety related to intimacy (Carroll, Rueger, Foy, & Donahoe, 1985; Riggs, Byrne, Weathers, & Litz, 1998). In a recent longitudinal cohort study of Iraq/Afghanistan war veterans, interpersonal relationship problems outpaced the occurrence of individual mental health problems by at least twice the rate (Milliken, Auchterlonie, & Hoge, 2007).

The health of intimate relationships plays a role not only as a presenting problem but also as a factor in treatment engagement. Recent research with service members returning from Iraq and Afghanistan suggests that strong intimate relationships are associated with higher rates of treatment engagement. In their large longitudinal study of male National Guard soldiers and their intimate female partners, Meis, Barry, Kehle, Erbes, and Polusny (2010) found that soldiers with the most satisfied intimate relationships were the most likely to engage in individual mental health treatment.

An important question to ask is whether individuals with traumatic stress-related problems want their loved ones involved in their therapy. At least one study indicates they do. Batten and colleagues (2009) found that more than 80% of the veterans in their outpatient U.S. Department of Veterans Affairs (VA) PTSD program desired their family members to be more involved in their treatment. They also found that 66% of the veterans wanted help to improve their communication skills with family members, which is a major focus of CBCT for PTSD. In addition, there have been consistent referrals to treatment programs situated in different settings offering

CBCT for PTSD. Clinicians practicing CBCT for PTSD have informed us of their ample referrals when they started offering the therapy.

Once engaged in therapy, retention and adherence to the interventions are crucial. Existing individual evidence-based psychotherapies for PTSD, such as prolonged exposure (Foa et al., 2007) and cognitive processing therapy (Resick et al., 2008), with their focus on direct confrontation of traumatic material, are potent therapies. However, there are a number of clients who do not complete them or only partially respond to treatment. A meta-analysis of randomized controlled psychotherapy trials for PTSD found that the average dropout rate from trauma-focused treatment is greater than 25% (Hembree et al., 2003); dropout rates from these therapies in clinical settings are generally higher (Pitman et al., 1996). The current dropout rate for CBCT for PTSD in our trials is about 15%, which we attribute to patients' having more social support while undertaking trauma-focused treatment, loved ones' knowledge and support of the treatment rationale, and diminished stress in the patients' interpersonal environments while participating in the therapy.

Individuals who complete an existing evidence-based psychotherapy for PTSD are likely to have symptom improvements. Randomized clinical trials demonstrate a remission rate of approximately 66% treatment completers (see, e.g., Bradley, Greene, Russ, Dutra, & Westen, 2005). These are impressive results compared with those for many other mental health conditions. However, this means that 33% of participants, who are sufficiently motivated to enter these trials and complete treatment, nevertheless still have a PTSD diagnosis at treatment end. There is clearly room for innovative therapies that can bridge this gap in success, increasing the number of patients who experience remission in their PTSD diagnosis upon completion of treatment. Incorporating significant others into PTSD treatment is one such innovation.

When armed with proper psychoeducation and skills, loved ones can be champions for the therapy and for interventions that are often the antithesis of what an individual with traumatic stress-related problems wants to do (i.e., to avoid). However, in the absence of understanding of how avoidance maintains PTSD and intimate relationship problems, for example, loved ones may unwittingly reinforce symptoms. Current evidence-based interventions for PTSD involve facing memories or current-day reminders of traumatic events. As we discuss in Chapter 2 regarding conceptualizing PTSD in a dyadic relationship, many loved ones "protect" the person with traumatic stress-related symptoms from the distress caused by facing these triggers. On the basis of our experience, we believe that these individuals, although usually well meaning, functionally collude in their loved one's cognitive, behavioral, and emotional avoidance, on which posttraumatic stress problems thrive. We have labeled these types of behaviors as "accommodation" to the symptoms because they serve to maintain the individual problems and make space in the relationship for the symptoms to exist. With the skills and education that CBCT for PTSD offers, couples work together to overcome this avoidance, which maintains or even increases the posttraumatic problems, and this sense of togetherness can then serve as an important motivator for patients engage in the hard work of therapy. As one of our clients stated, "What I won't do for myself, I'll do for my family."

We have also had cases in which loved ones were not privy to the rationale for individual trauma-focused CBT for PTSD and were upset by the interventions. Some even encouraged behaviors that ran in opposition to the interventions. In one case a wife called to ask, "Why, Dr. Monson, after all of these years of me helping to 'button him up,' are you trying to unhinge him?" In another case, a client reported in session that her partner had offered her a glass of wine before she was to listen to an audiotaped account of her trauma memory at home, stating, "He thought it would chill me out, and it did." Again, we presume that most significant others are acting with the best of intentions, albeit misguided. Including significant others in the treatment of clients' posttraumatic problems can be beneficial not only in improving symptom-level outcomes but, as we discuss next, also for the loved ones themselves and their relationships.

### *Efficacy of CBCT for PTSD: Getting Three-for-One Benefits*

Perhaps the most important reason for considering conjoint therapy for PTSD is that you can simultaneously achieve benefits for (1) the person diagnosed with PTSD, (2) his or her loved one, and (3) their relationship. Our initial test of the therapy showing this three-for-one benefit was with romantic couples, including seven male Vietnam War veterans with PTSD and their wives (Monson, Schnurr, Stevens, & Guthrie, 2004). We found significant and large effect size improvements in clinicians' and partners' ratings of veterans' PTSD symptoms from pre- to posttreatment. The veterans reported moderate improvements in PTSD and statistically significant, large improvements in depression, anxiety, and social functioning. Wives reported large effect size improvements in relationship satisfaction, general anxiety, and social functioning (Monson, Stevens, & Schnurr, 2005).

We have since applied the therapy to a range of couples and trauma survivors diagnosed with PTSD. A recent uncontrolled study (Monson et al., 2011) revealed clinically significant improvements in clinicians', patients', and partners' ratings of patients' PTSD symptoms, and five of the six patients who completed treatment no longer carried a PTSD diagnosis by the end of the therapy. Three of the four couples who presented as distressed before treatment were satisfied after treatment, and partners reported significant improvements in their relationship satisfaction. In addition, patients reported large effect size improvements in depression and state anger symptoms, and partners reported large and significant improvements in their ability to express anger.

We are currently completing a randomized controlled trial of the therapy compared with treatment as usual in a diverse sample of couples and with survivors of different types of trauma. The available results from this trial show even stronger outcomes than those previously found. These results have been replicated in several cases outside of our research clinics as well (Schumm, Fredman, Monson, & Chard, 2012).

## Cognitive-Behavioral Interpersonal Theory Underlying CBCT for PTSD

Understanding the theoretical model upon which CBCT for PTSD was built is critical to case conceptualization and the successful implementation of this protocol-driven intervention. The more you understand the cognitive, behavioral, and emotional factors that interact to maintain traumatic stress-related problems and relationship difficulties, the better able you will be to think broadly and flexibly about how to implement the treatment with a given dyad while staying true to the treatment protocol. Here we discuss traumatic stress-related symptoms and associated relationship problems and describe how the different components of CBCT for PTSD target these difficulties. The descriptions are not exhaustive but rather illustrative examples;

the vast range of symptom presentations and complex manifestations within different intimate relationships preclude description here.

The art of delivering this manualized treatment relies on the ability to deliver the essential ingredients of the therapy as prescribed while simultaneously considering how a variety of thoughts, feelings, and behaviors on the part of each partner interact to maintain the problems and associated relationship difficulties and then addressing them in the context of the particular couple. For instance, we assert that there are as many ways for individuals and couples to avoid trauma-related material as there are people struggling with posttraumatic sequelae. Your ability to conceptualize these behaviors within an interpersonal, cognitive-behavioral framework and then translate this understanding into a curious and nonjudgmental inquiry about the potential function of these behaviors will ultimately facilitate clients' recovery from PTSD and relationship problems.

## PTSD as a Disorder of Impeded Recovery

CBCT for PTSD is based on a recovery model of traumatic stress-related problems. In this approach to PTSD, symptoms are not considered as developing over time, like many other mental health conditions that have early warning signs or a prodromal phase (e.g., depression, schizophrenia). Rather, prospective studies indicate that, in the acute aftermath of exposure to a traumatic event, most individuals will have an assortment of symptoms later identified as PTSD symptoms if they have lasted the 1 month required by the *Diagnostic and Statistical Manual of Mental Disorders* (DSM). With time, most people will experience abatement in their symptoms, and they will naturally "recover" without intervention (Ehlers, Mayou, & Bryant, 1998; Riggs, Rothbaum, & Foa, 1995; Rothbaum, Foa, Riggs, & Murdock, 1992). The evidence suggests that delayed-onset cases of PTSD are most generally characterized by subthreshold diagnoses at prior evaluations (Bryant & Harvey, 2002; Buckley, Blanchard, & Hickling, 1996; Ehlers et al., 1998).

Epidemiological data regarding trauma exposure and subsequent PTSD diagnosis also illustrate this point regarding natural recovery. As mentioned, approximately 75% of North Americans will be exposed to traumatic stressors (Kessler et al., 1995; Van Ameringen, Mancini, Patterson, & Boyle, 2008). However, only about 5% of men and 10% of women will be diagnosed with PTSD in their lifetime, indicating that a substantial majority have natural remission of their symptoms after exposure. When implementing CBCT for PTSD, you should think about what got in the way, or impeded, that natural recovery process.

The notion of impeded recovery is integral to the rationale for CBCT for PTSD and, as such, is built into the description of the therapy course for therapists and clients alike. More specifically, we chose the acronym R.E.S.U.M.E. Living to characterize the three phases of the therapy (discussed later) and convey its recovery orientation and to imbue hope for improvements in traumatic stress symptoms, relationship problems, and quality of life more broadly.

In prior work, we have outlined a cognitive-behavioral interpersonal theory of PTSD (Monson, Fredman, & Dekel, 2010; Monson, Fredman, Dekel, & Macdonald, in press). Translating this theory into the interventions that make up CBCT for PTSD, traumatic stress-related problems are postulated to result from behavioral, cognitive, and emotional factors that interact within each individual and also between members of a couple. These interacting systems simultaneously create a shared relationship milieu that, in turn, feeds back on the individuals

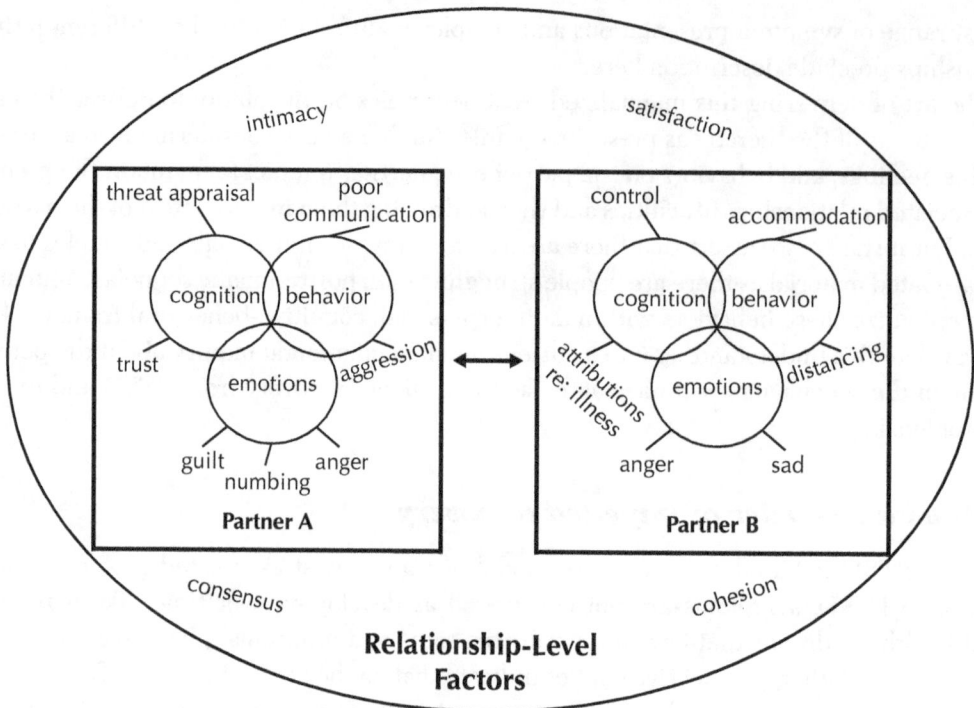

**FIGURE 1.** Example of interacting cognitive, behavioral, and emotional factors within and between partners and the influence on and by relationship factors (Monson et al., 2010).

existing within that milieu (see Figure 1 for examples of factors). These factors are postulated to impede the natural trajectory toward recovery. Implicated behavioral mechanisms include communication deficits and various types of avoidance. Cognitive mechanisms involve problematic appraisals of the event and related conclusions drawn in the here and now that emanate from those appraisals. Emotional mechanisms include disturbances in a range of emotions and in the processes that govern these emotions (i.e., identifying, experiencing, sharing).

## *Behavioral Mechanisms*

In behavioral models of PTSD, classical conditioning accounts for the associations between certain stimuli and physiological and psychological distress when confronted with the stimuli. For example, we have had cases in which fireworks provoked arousal for combat veterans because the sights and loud, unexpected noises reminded them of war zone explosions to which they were exposed. In another case, the sight of an automated teller machine (ATM) provoked distress in a client who was robbed at knifepoint during an ATM transaction. For a rape victim whom we treated, the smell of spearmint gum was a source of distress because her attacker was chewing that flavor of gum at the time of the assault. In these cases, a previously neutral stimulus (e.g., loud noise, ATM, spearmint gum) took on distressing properties because it was paired in time with the traumatic event.

Operant conditioning, and specifically the negatively reinforcing value of avoiding distressing internal and external reminders, accounts for the maintenance of the distress response when confronted with traumatic material (Mowrer, 1960). That is, when traumatized individuals avoid people, places, situations, or other stimuli that remind them of the traumatic event(s), they feel less distressed or uncomfortable in the moment and, therefore, are more likely to keep avoiding over time. As a result, they are denied the opportunity for new associations to develop and to learn that they are, in fact, safe in the present. Through these processes, avoidance provides short-term relief but paradoxical long-term maintenance, or even exacerbation, of the distress.

When conceptualizing avoidance within CBCT for PTSD, it is important to consider a broad range of behaviors that can strengthen the association between trauma stimuli and distress. These include the classic behavioral avoidance and emotional numbing symptoms. However, there are behaviors beyond these traditional symptoms that can serve an avoidance function. Some of these behaviors are more active in nature, while others are more indirect or passive. Examples of active avoidance include alcohol or other substance use, angry outbursts to dissuade others from discussing particular topics, self-harm, workaholism, electronic gaming, sex, safety behaviors (e.g., scanning/patrolling areas), pornography, nonattendance at sessions, and noncompletion of out-of-session assignments. Other, more passive behaviors that can serve an avoidance function include dissociation, social withdrawal, somatic complaints, skirting difficult topics, and sleeping. Any behavior that serves to minimize exposure to trauma reminders or memories may be avoidance. One question to consider in monitoring for avoidance is "If not for the traumatic event, would the person be engaging in (or not engaging in) the behavior?"

At the dyadic level, significant others' well-intended caretaking or "accommodation" behaviors—efforts to assuage the distress of affected family members by minimizing their loved one's exposure to stimuli that he or she finds aversive—can also serve to promote or maintain avoidant behavior. For example, family members of a motor vehicle accident survivor may drive him everywhere because of his anxiety at the mere thought of driving a car. Likewise, a combat veteran and his partner may avoid crowded venues, such as restaurants, theaters, or concerts, because, as targets of bombings during his deployment, they serve as trauma-related triggers. Rape survivors and their loved ones might avoid sexual intimacy in general or particular sexual positions or behaviors because they are reminiscent of the assault. Loved ones can also accommodate the symptoms of PTSD by colluding in safety behaviors and by serving as safety signals in distressing situations. For example, partners may participate in excessively checking door and window locks, carry weapons at their partner's insistence, avoid certain highways when they drive, or agree to around-the-clock cell phone accessibility so that their PTSD+ loved one can call for safety reassurance. We have also had cases in which the presence of partners and children was used to manage distress in stressful environments (e.g., grocery stores, malls) by serving either as a form of reassurance or distraction.

Over time, avoidance leads to the unfortunate consequence of diminished relationship satisfaction because of less engagement in shared rewarding activities and restraints on partners' behaviors, feelings, and communication. Connecting around mutually satisfying events and experiences represents an important way for couples to nurture and invest in their relationships and to buffer against the effects of the inevitable ups and downs that characterize even healthy relationships. However, when couples are deprived of opportunities to connect as a result of behavioral avoidance, their relationships can become distressed because of the absence of positive interactions. These couples also become more attentive to their negative interactions, which contributes to relationship dissatisfaction (Epstein & Baucom, 2002).

Other behavioral mechanisms implicated in the cognitive-behavioral interpersonal theory of PTSD are poor communication and conflict management skills. Individuals with PTSD display communication skills deficits (Nezu & Carnevale, 1987), which may be a risk factor or consequence of the disorder. Hyperarousal symptoms such as anger/irritability, hypervigilance, and sleeplessness fuel these deficits and contribute to negative interpersonal interactions, which can be characterized by verbal and physical aggression (Taft, Vogt, Marshall, Panuzio, & Niles, 2007; Taft et al., 2009). Problematic communication is characteristic of unhappy couples, and communication problems are one of the most commonly reported reasons why couples seek therapy (Geiss & O'Leary, 1981). Deficits in communication skills, coupled with behavioral constriction, avoidance, and emotional numbing, can also lead to problems with emotional intimacy. Deficits in communication skills and diminished emotional intimacy can also decrease the likelihood of trauma disclosure. As discussed shortly, trauma disclosure in an encouraging and supportive environment can lead to the development of a more cogent trauma narrative and emotional processing of traumatic memories.

## Cognitive Mechanisms

There are related cognitive thematic content and processes that are theorized to account for the association between individual posttraumatic stress and close relationship problems. A primary barrier to trauma recovery is maladaptive appraisals about the traumatic event(s). There are a variety of different ways in which individuals and significant others can maladaptively appraise traumatic events that lead to posttraumatic symptomatology and intimate relationship problems. These barriers include a variety of social-cognitive constructs, including hindsight bias and its derivatives (e.g., "undoing" the event by thinking about alternative actions that may have prevented the event; "happily-ever-after" thinking that an alternative action would have led to a positive outcome), just-world thinking (the belief that good things happen to good people and bad things happen to bad people), and actor–observer biases (i.e., not fully appreciating the situational variables that affect behavior; making characterological attributions about situationally influenced behavior). Examples of these misappraisals include the rape victim who believes she should have fought back because it would have prevented the rape and the combat medic who believes he failed to prevent his comrade's death despite a lack of knowledge and tools to perform surgery on the battlefield. Significant others, including therapists, can also fall prey to these appraisal errors and thereby influence trauma survivors' appraisals about trauma events. Examples of maladaptive attributions sometimes held by loved ones include victim-blaming attributions (e.g., "You shouldn't have worn that outfit," "If you hadn't have drunk alcohol . . . ," and "You drove unsafe") and characterological attributions about those involved in traumatic events (e.g., describing combat veterans as "baby killers" and sexual assault victims as "sluts" or "provocative"). These appraisal barriers to recovery are described in more depth in Sessions 8 and 9. In general, these barriers can be conceptualized as efforts to exert predictability and control over the events by clients, loved ones, and therapists. Yet they leave the traumatized person with unprocessed traumatic material and the related symptoms.

Problematic appraisals about traumatic events can lead to overgeneralized maladaptive beliefs about the self, others, and the world after traumatization. Borrowing from earlier work by McCann and Pearlman (1990), and consistent with content found in cognitive processing therapy (Resick et al., 2008), beliefs about trust, power, and intimacy are affected by traumatization.

For example, prior positive beliefs in these areas may be challenged by traumatization (e.g., "I thought I could trust my judgment and the person who assaulted me") or prior negative beliefs could be seemingly confirmed (e.g., "I knew men could not be trusted"). These beliefs are extremely pertinent to close relationship functioning. Consider an incest survivor who believes she will be betrayed again if she were to become emotionally vulnerable with another person. As a consequence of her belief, she avoids emotional intimacy with her partner and lashes out preemptively in an effort to protect herself before she can be hurt again. Other couples we have worked with have been characterized by overly controlling behaviors on the part of the traumatized individual as a result of the belief that the world in general was an unsafe place. For example, some combat veterans have demanded to know where their partners and children were at all times with the belief that they could protect them from perceived harm by untrustworthy others.

In addition to cognitive content that is disturbed with traumatization, there are cognitive process disturbances associated with PTSD, including attention/concentration deficits and selective attention to negativity (Vasterling & Brewin, 2005). Not uncommonly, selective attention to threat extends to the perceptions of the partner's behaviors, such as the suspicion that the partner's intentions toward the traumatized individual are negative. For instance, when asked by his wife where he was earlier in the day, the traumatized individual could construe this as an accusation that he was having an extramarital affair. Selective attention to negative relationship behaviors, negative attributions for each other's behaviors, and negative assumptions and expectancies about each other also characterize couples experiencing relationship distress more generally (Epstein & Baucom, 2002). Thus, the tendency among couples in which at least one partner has PTSD to view each other as a source of threat is similar to that observed in other distressed couples and tends to be amplified in the presence of PTSD.

In addition to those who have been directly traumatized, significant others can hold maladaptive beliefs that interfere with therapy and, consequently, trauma recovery. For instance, a combat veteran client was dissuaded by his wife from approaching safe places and situations that caused him anxiety (e.g., the mall, grocery store) because of her belief that even mild stress would cause her husband to suffer a heart attack. Because of his wife's maladaptive cognition and related protective behavior, the veteran had not had the opportunity to place himself in anxiety-provoking situations and learn that he was actually safe. With cognitive interventions, however, the wife was able to facilitate her husband's approach of these safe situations, with the realization that he might be more at risk for cardiovascular problems resulting from chronic PTSD than with prescribed and planned approaches to trauma-related stimuli like a crowded mall.

## *Emotional Mechanisms*

Although PTSD has been defined as an anxiety disorder within the current DSM classification system, research has shown that the emotional disturbances associated with traumatization extend beyond anxiety. For instance, there is strong evidence that individuals with PTSD experience disruption in a range of emotions in addition to fear, such as guilt, shame, anger, grief, and sadness (e.g., Kubany & Watson, 2002; Novaco & Chemtob, 2002). Moreover, avoidance can generalize to the experience and expression of emotions more generally in PTSD (Boeschen, Koss, Figueredo, & Coan, 2001; Morina, Stangier, & Risch, 2008). Emotional process disturbances such as alexithymia and difficulty identifying and expressing emotions have also been associated with PTSD (Price, Monson, Callahan, & Rodriguez, 2006).

These emotional content and process disturbances are suspected to contribute to emotional communication deficits and their related relationship impairments, such as an inability to relate on an emotionally intimate level. As we discuss in Session 4, emotions are the "glue" that hold couples together. With the exception of hostility, the expression of emotions enhances emotional intimacy regardless of the valence of the emotion that is shared (i.e., whether the emotion is positive or negative). Alexithymia and other difficulties labeling emotions interfere with traumatized individuals' ability to name and share their emotions with others and can be especially deleterious to relationship satisfaction. Indeed, research has shown that it is the emotional numbing symptoms of PTSD that are most strongly associated with lower relationship satisfaction (Riggs et al., 1998) and are not as responsive to existing individual evidence-based therapies for PTSD (Asmundson, Stapleton, & Taylor, 2004).

## Specific Mechanisms of PTSD and Relationship Problems Targeted in CBCT for PTSD

To address the interacting behavioral, cognitive, and emotional processes postulated to underlie PTSD and associated relationship problems, CBCT for PTSD consists of 15 sessions organized into three phases that build upon one another. The acronym R.E.S.U.M.E. Living was chosen to reflect these sequential phases and the recovery-focused nature of the therapy for therapists and clients alike:

R = *Rationale* for Treatment  
E = *Education* about PTSD and Relationships } Phase 1

S = *Satisfaction* Enhancement  
U = *Undermining* Avoidance } Phase 2

M = *Making Meaning* of the Trauma(s)  
E = *End* of Therapy—commitment to ongoing betterment } Phase 3  
Living

Table 1 presents an overview of the sessions of CBCT for PTSD.

### Phase 1. Rationale for Treatment and Education about PTSD and Relationships (Sessions 1–2)

In this phase, couples receive a rationale for treatment, an overview of the protocol, and psychoeducation about the reciprocal influences of PTSD symptoms and relationship adjustment, including an explanation of how avoidance, emotional numbing, and maladaptive thinking maintain both PTSD and relationship difficulties. At the end of Session 1, they are asked (1) to catch each other doing nice things in order to promote positivity in their relationship and decrease selective attention to negative relationship behaviors and (2) to read a psychoeducational handout on the association between PTSD symptoms and relationship behaviors. Both

**TABLE 1. Overview of CBCT for PTSD**

R.E.S.U.M.E. Living

**Phase 1. Rationale for Treatment and Education about PTSD and Relationships**

Session 1. Introduction to Treatment
Session 2. Safety Building

**Phase 2. Satisfaction Enhancement and Undermining Avoidance**

Session 3. Listening and Approaching
Session 4. Sharing Thoughts and Feelings: Emphasis on *Feelings*
Session 5. Sharing Thoughts and Feelings: Emphasis on *Thoughts*
Session 6. Getting U.N.S.T.U.C.K.
Session 7. Problem Solving to Shrink PTSD

**Phase 3. Making Meaning of the Trauma(s) and End of Therapy**

Session 8. Acceptance
Session 9. Blame
Session 10. Trust
Session 11. Control
Session 12. Emotional Closeness
Session 13. Physical Closeness
Session 14. Posttraumatic Growth
Session 15. Review and Reinforcement of Treatment Gains

partners are also asked to complete the Trauma Impact Questions-I (TIQ-I); see Part II, Session 1, Handout 1.5), which is designed to elicit their thoughts about how PTSD has affected their relationship and the perceived causes of the traumatic event(s) as well as their thoughts about themselves, each other, and the world in general in the areas of trust, control, emotional closeness, and physical closeness. These are then shared and read aloud at the next session. In Session 2, in addition to reviewing the partners' responses on the TIQ-I, the couple is educated about how PTSD contributes to a range of aggressive behaviors because of dysregulation in the fight–flight–freeze system, and they learn strategies to facilitate a shared sense of safety, such as recognizing early warning signs of anger, slowed breathing, and time-out conflict management strategies. To increase the likelihood of skill use outside of the session, the couple has the opportunity to practice slowed breathing and the time-out technique during the session.

## Phase 2. Satisfaction Enhancement and Undermining Avoidance (Sessions 3–7)

In Phase 2, couples learn about the insidious role of avoidance in maintaining both PTSD and relationship problems and are taught communication skills to address both. Enhanced dyadic communication is used as an antidote to PTSD-related emotional numbing and avoidance and as a means of increasing emotional intimacy. In Session 3, couples use the communication skill of reflective listening to begin generating a list of people, places, situations, and feelings that they have avoided as a couple as a result of PTSD. Starting in Session 4 and continuing through the rest of the therapy, this "avoidance" list becomes their "approach" list, and ideographically programmed, trauma-relevant *in vivo* approach assignments from the approach list are completed after each session in a graduated manner. Special attention is paid to the selection of *in vivo* approach activities that will address behavioral and experiential avoidance and concurrently double as shared rewarding activities. For example, a couple who has avoided restaurants because crowded places serve as a trigger for the PTSD-identified partner would first be asked to go the restaurant during the week in the early afternoon when it is unlikely to be crowded, then go on a weeknight evening, and ultimately to go on a Saturday night while the patient sits with his or her back against the wall in order to decrease PTSD-related hypervigilance. These exercises are similar to *in vivo* exposures completed in the context of prolonged exposure (Foa et al., 2007). However, they differ in that no formal SUDS (Subjective Units of Distress Scale) ratings are made, as is typically done in the treatment of anxiety disorders. In addition, the couple's relationship is the unit of intervention rather than the patient and his or her disorder only. Consequently, both partners participate in the exercise instead of the non-PTSD partner serving as a surrogate therapist or coach.

Communication skills presented and practiced in each session build on each other over several sessions to help the couple identify and share their feelings and notice the way that their thoughts influence their feelings and behaviors. For example, in Session 4, couples learn the skill of channel checking to differentiate between conversations focused on sharing thoughts and feelings versus trying to solve a problem or make a decision. They then use reflective listening skills to discuss the feelings they each have about the role of PTSD in their relationship (e.g., angry, sad) and, in Session 5, use the reflective listening skills to identify and share thoughts and related feelings that they have as a result of PTSD (e.g., "PTSD makes me think that I can't trust anybody, and that makes me feel sad and angry"). In Session 6, the couple learns a dyadic cognitive intervention process that they use together to increase flexibility in thinking and to challenge cognitions that maintain both PTSD and relationship problems (e.g., "If I go to the movies with Jake, I will be attacked"). Consistent with the notion that the couple is together identifying and modifying these maladaptive thoughts, or "stuck points," related to traumatization, the steps of the process are summarized in the acronym U.N.S.T.U.C.K.:

- Unified and curious as a couple as you join together in collaborative empiricism.
- Notice and share thoughts (e.g., "If I go to the movies with Jake, I will be attacked," with a corresponding feeling of fear).
- (Brain)Storm alternative thoughts or interpretations, no matter how implausible they might seem initially (e.g., "Although it's possible that something bad could happen, it's extremely unlikely," "My PTSD makes me exaggerate the risk that we could be hurt at the movies").
- Test the thoughts (i.e., consider the evidence for and against each alternative thought generated; e.g., "I used to go the movies, and nothing bad ever happened," "I don't know anyone who's ever been attacked at a movie," "There will be a lot of people around, so it's unlikely that someone could actually hurt us if someone did something dangerous")
- Use the most balanced or reasonable thought(s) (e.g., "Although it's possible that something bad could happen, it's extremely unlikely").

- Changes in emotions and behaviors that result from the new thought(s) (e.g., less scared, less avoidant of going to crowded places).
- Keep practicing by generating specific behavior(s) that will reinforce this new way of thinking (e.g., schedule a date on Saturday night and go to the movie theater for a matinee).

In Session 7, the couple learns the skill of problem solving to decide how they will continue to "shrink" the role of PTSD in their relationship by collaboratively addressing PTSD-related avoidance, and they practice this skill in session by determining their next *in vivo* approach activity. For example, in the case described previously, the couple might use their problem-solving skills to decide which theater they will go to, when they will go, what movie they will see, and what they will do if one or both of them feels anxious before or during the exercise.

## *Phase 3. Making Meaning of the Trauma(s) and End of Therapy (Sessions 8–14)*

The final phase of therapy capitalizes on the couple's improved communication skills and their new tendency to approach rather than avoid by examining trauma-related beliefs that they may each hold that contribute to PTSD symptoms and relationship problems. Discussions focus directly on the resolution of problematic appraisals of the trauma and then proceed to specific problematic core beliefs that have been impacted by the event and maintain PTSD and relationship difficulties. These domains include trust, control, emotional closeness, and physical intimacy. Sessions are sequenced in Phase 3 with a focus on appraisals specific to the trauma first because more accurate appraisal of the traumatic event(s) should have robust and cascading effects on present- and future-oriented beliefs that have been affected by (mis-)appraisals of traumatic events. When progressing to the core areas, the therapist guides the couple to investigate how the traumatic event has influenced thoughts in each core area and to challenge any appraisals that influence current-day individual and relationship functioning. For instance, we have worked with many rape survivors who have had the thought "I should have known that he was going to rape me and could have prevented this" or "I should have fought back harder." As a result, they harbored current-day beliefs that they could not trust their own judgment in the here and now and consequently relied on their partners to make all decisions for fear that any decision they made would result in danger, which, in turn, contributed to their partners feeling burdened and frustrated. We have seen many cases in which the couple successfully used the U.N.S.T.U.C.K. process to notice and challenge these thoughts by taking more a contextualized view of the event and considered alternatives to PTSD-related cognitions, such as "The rapist had the element of surprise on his side, and I had no way of predicting that this would happen" or "If I had fought back, I might have gotten hurt worse or been killed." Once the survivor learned to accurately place blame with the rapist rather than herself, the thinking frequently shifted from presently believing that she could not trust her own judgment to believing that she could rely on her ability to make good decisions to keep herself safe in many, but not all, situations. We have seen similar shifts in thinking with combat veterans. With the help of their partner's being curious and asking questions, they were able to challenge historical misappraisals of traumatic events (e.g., "I should have known an IED [improvised explosive device] was about to go off" to "There's no way that I could have known there was an IED. They were deliberately placed so that we would be unable to predict the explosions"). The veterans experienced corresponding shifts in current-day thinking (e.g., "I have to try to control everything to prevent bad things from happening to me or my partner" to "I can control some, but not all, things in my life, and it is ultimately better for my relationship for me to share control with my partner than to try to control all aspects of our relationship in an attempt to keep us safe"). Treatment culminates with a discussion of the potential for benefit finding and posttraumatic growth and ends with a review of gains made in therapy and challenges expected in the future.

We have found processing appraisals and the consequent meaning of traumatic events in an interpersonal context to be very powerful in terms of not only accelerated healing and reduction of symptoms but also increasing closeness and deepening close relationships. Significant others often provide alternative explanations for traumatic events, support the survivor in confronting the trauma memory to do the reappraisal work, and help the survivor practice new ways of making sense of the traumatic experiences and the consequences of those experiences in the interpersonal interactions. Consistent with the literature on self-disclosure about traumatic events and relationship functioning (Koenen, Stellman, Stellman, & Sommer, 2003; Solomon, Dekel, & Zerach, 2008), it is our experience that this type of work increases intimacy in the couple beyond that achieved with more traditional couple therapy techniques and enhances understanding and empathy in the couple's relationship.

## *Important Therapeutic Assumptions*

CBCT for PTSD is based on several assumptions. First, and consistent with a family systems perspective, the nature of the problem is the way that the couple relates around the posttrauma sequelae and not something inherently pathological in the partner diagnosed with PTSD. Accordingly, the treatment is disorder specific, meaning that the targets of intervention are the interactions within the couple; and the patient, in this case, is the couple's relationship vis-à-vis the PTSD. This is in contrast to partner-assisted models of couple/family-based treatments for individual psychopathology in which the partner functions as a coach or surrogate therapist (Baucom, Shoham, Mueser, Daiuto, & Stickle, 1998). Second, we presume that individuals with PTSD will have significant others with their own mental health issues, whether by virtue of assortative mating (Merikangas, 1982; i.e., the tendency to partner with someone similar to oneself) or as a consequence of living with someone with untreated PTSD. The third assumption is that PTSD and relationship problems are reciprocally related. That is, we do not presume that PTSD necessarily causes relationship problems or that relationship problems cause PTSD. Rather, there is a bidirectional association in which each influences the other, which is why an intervention that addresses both concurrently is indicated. Last, following a manualized treatment such as CBCT for PTSD does not replace the need for good nonspecific therapy skills, such as warmth and empathy. Many of the patients and significant others whom we see have been struggling with PTSD and its effects for years and come to us feeling discouraged and demoralized, both about the possibility of recovery from PTSD and the thought of improving the relationship. Providing a compelling rationale for treatment and skill use in the context of an encouraging and collaborative therapeutic relationship can be a powerful motivator for change, especially given that we are asking both members of the couples to try a new way of relating to each other specifically and to others more generally.

## Therapist Preparation

Any provider sanctioned to provide psychotherapy, or in training and supervised by someone who is sanctioned to provide psychotherapy, is eligible to deliver CBCT for PTSD. With regard to preferable clinical experience, we have found that most clinicians do not have experience providing conjoint therapy for specific mental health conditions. The providers who we train often either have experience providing generic couple/family therapy or individual/group therapy for PTSD, and those therapies may or may not be evidence based. Because we have created a treatment that capitalizes on evidence-based interventions in each area, clinicians with experience in CBT for either couple distress or PTSD tend to find ease in transitioning to provide CBCT for PTSD. For example, those practitioners using couple behavioral therapy will find the communication skills training familiar; those using exposure-based therapies for PTSD will recognize the use of *in vivo* exposure exercises; and those practicing cognitive therapies for PTSD and/or relationship distress can draw on their Socratic dialogue skills. To facilitate confidence and competence in delivering the interventions, we provide a detailed set of session-by-session instructions later in this volume. In addition, we have a program that offers a variety of supports to providers to facilitate their delivery of the therapy. These supports include workshop training, group teleconsultation, and expert review of audio-recorded therapy sessions for fidelity to the model. Clinicians have the option of achieving certification in CBCT for PTSD. More information regarding our training program can be found at *www.coupletherapyforptsd.com*.

Successful implementation of a manualized therapy involves the clinician's employing the essential but nonspecific ingredients of any efficacious psychotherapy. These ingredients include building a solid working alliance with the couple based on empathy, genuineness, warmth, and support. Consistent with our attention to these key ingredients, we evaluate the presence of them and therapist competence in delivering them when we rate clinicians' adherence and competence in delivering CBCT for PTSD.

## Considerations in Implementing CBCT for PTSD

### Piecemeal versus Protocol Implementation

CBCT for PTSD has been designed and tested to be 15 sessions of 75 minutes. It may be tempting to treat the protocol as a guide for conducting treatment with couples in which at least one partner has been traumatized, picking and choosing interventions or allowing the treatment to expand to an undetermined number of sessions. We caution against the use of the protocol in this way. First, the interventions were developed to be sequentially delivered. Even in couples with no significant relationship distress (likely the exception rather than the rule given the research on relationship distress and PTSD; Taft, Watkins, Stafford, Street, & Monson, 2011), the interventions designed to enhance relationship functioning in Phases 1 and 2 can improve the dyadic milieu in which the individuals exist. Perhaps more importantly, distressed and nondistressed couples alike can interact in ways that advertently and inadvertently contribute to avoidance. Second, because of trauma-related distress and the related avoidance hallmark to PTSD, most people who have it will procrastinate to change. Thus, we believe that an active ingredient of the therapy is its time-limited and structured nature. We support contracting to conduct the therapy as designed, evaluating the progress of the individuals and couples throughout and especially at the end, and then recontracting for an episode of goal-driven therapy at the conclusion of the therapy if necessary. Related to this last point, we encourage therapists to give the couple or each individual in the couple a break from therapy that is at least 1 month long (preferably longer) to determine whether further changes occur or are maintained before immediately pursuing another episode of care. Follow-up assessments from PTSD treatment studies, including CBCT for PTSD, suggest maintained gains or even further improvements in symptoms and functioning (e.g., Resick, Williams, Suvak, Monson, & Gradus, 2012). Thus, therapists are urged to allow for a break or "holiday" from treatment to determine the longer term effects of therapy and whether additional sessions are indicated.

## Pacing Therapy Sessions

A key to delivering manualized therapies successfully, in general, is pacing the delivery of interventions within each session. After the first session, in which the therapist speaks relatively more compared with future sessions in order to provide psychoeducation about the symptoms of PTSD in an interpersonal context and the rationale for the therapy, the therapist is urged to consider the following suggested time frames in pacing each of the 75-minute therapy sessions (see Figure 2). Approximately 30 minutes should be spent reviewing the couple's out-of-session assignment (OOSA) and/or troubleshooting difficulties in completing the OOSAs. Approximately 10 minutes is then spent teaching new skills or introducing specific content, depending on the session. Consistent with the importance of experiential exercises in couple/family therapies, we suggest that approximately 25 minutes of the session be spent practicing the new skill or focusing the couple on interacting about the new content introduced in the session. The balance of the session is spent introducing the next OOSA to the couple (approximately 5 minutes) and doing a check-out (approximately 5 minutes) from the session. The check-out consists of inquiring of the couple what they took from the session, reinforcing any learning that the therapist observed in the session, and emotionally containing or sending the couple out on a positive note as they leave the session.

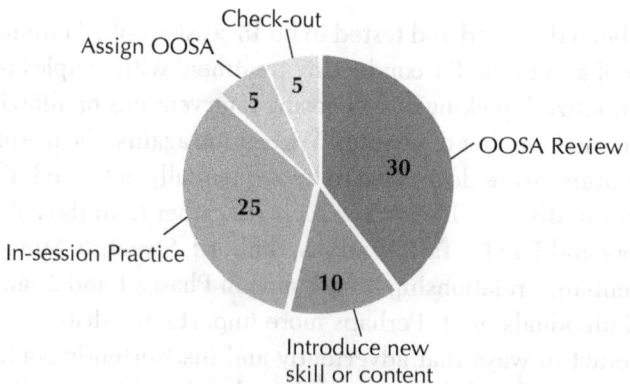

**FIGURE 2.** Pacing of CBCT for PTSD sessions beginning with Session 2 (numbers indicate minutes).

## *Managing Clients' Nonadherence to the Protocol*

One of the most important skills for a psychotherapist delivering skills-focused interventions is the management of clients' nonadherence with prescribed interventions. (Note that we use the term *adherence* rather than *compliance* to convey the shared responsibility between the couple and therapist to increase the likelihood of completing the interventions and choice on the part of the couple to engage in the interventions.) We recommend preempting nonadherence whenever possible, and this begins at the point of treatment contracting. As discussed further in Chapter 2, we recommend reviewing couples' prior experiences with psychotherapy to determine the number and types that they have pursued to improve their relationship and to assess their experience with therapies that require work outside of session. In contracting for a course of CBCT for PTSD, it is important that both members of the couple are fully informed about the expectation of completing tasks outside of session. We specifically introduce the value of "getting the interventions out of the therapy room and into their lives," noting the documented relationship between homework completion and treatment outcomes (Kazantzis, Deane, & Ronan, 2000; Kazantzis, Whittington, & Dattilio, 2010).

Laying a rationale for the OOSAs assigned at the end of each CBCT for PTSD session is an integral step to maximizing adherence. If a client does not understand the reason for an assignment, he or she is less likely to see it as important and tied to recovery. For example, in CBCT for PTSD, couples are assigned OOSAs related to decreasing avoidance and increasing the occurrence of shared, pleasurable events (i.e., approach assignments). If the couple does not understand the role of avoidance in maintaining PTSD and relationship problems, they are not likely to engage in behaviors that cause distress in the short term for longer term benefits. After assigning an OOSA, it is useful to ask the couple why you are asking them to engage in particular tasks in order to gauge their understanding of the rationale for completion and to assess whether both of them seem to understand and buy into it. This gives you an opportunity to correct any misunderstandings about the assignment or the reasons for asking them to do it. We also let the couple know that we will begin the next session with a review of the work that they have done outside of session.

To promote OOSA adherence and decrease the likelihood of spending too much time on the couple's most recent conflict, the clinician should begin each session with an inquiry about how the OOSAs went. This will help focus the session and reinforce the value placed on OOSA completion. The therapist should be sure to review the couple's written work and praise them for any efforts, even if small in nature, and determine with the couple any areas in need of troubleshooting to improve the efficacy of the interventions.

When nonadherence occurs, we recommend five steps to address it. The first is to determine what got in the way of completing the assignment. For example, did the couple not understand what they were asked to do (knowledge deficit)? Do they believe that PTSD and/or their relationship cannot improve (motivational deficit)? Both partners may have different barriers to completing the assignment, and each of their reasons should be elucidated in order to address adherence maximally. The second step is to inquire why they might choose to do the specific OOSAs. It is our experience that clinicians are prone to telling couples the value of doing the assignments when nonadherence occurs. Consistent with the curious spirit of the cognitive interventions making up CBCT for PTSD, we suggest that you become and remain very inquisitive with the couple about why they might choose to complete the OOSAs, even suggesting that they treat the assignments as experiments to see what might happen if they were to try them.

The third recommended step in addressing nonadherence is to do some work in session. To increase the likelihood of completion the first time or subsequent times that an assignment is made, it is recommended that the therapist do a bit of the work in session. For example, if the couple did not practice paraphrasing at least 5 minutes per day after Session 3, the therapist could ask the couple to practice the skill briefly in session with the therapist coaching. A key part of this recommendation is that the couple does only some, not all, of the work in session. Otherwise, the couple may rely on session time only to complete assignments.

The fourth step is to anticipate barriers and how to overcome them. When thinking about completing the work, what do the partners anticipate will get in the way? What will they do when that happens? After collecting this information, it is recommended that you get very specific about the "who, what, when, and where" of OOSA completion for the next time— the more concrete the better. The couple should consider who will prompt completion (taking turns is recommended to maintain a good balance of power between partners), what they will complete, when they will complete it, and where they will get it done. A concrete example is difficulty completing the OOSA approach assignment of riding public transportation. In session the therapist helps the couple determine which partner will initiate the actual ride, the form of transportation, the day and time it will happen, and the stop they will get on and off. The therapist reviews at the next session how the assignment went.

The final step in addressing nonadherence is to reassign the OOSA and move on to the next. It is important not only to reassign the OOSA not completed but also to assign the next set of OOSAs. This approach helps you to send a message of expected mastery—you believe that they can do the assignments and, therefore, you do not need to hold them up until they "get it." It also helps you to avoid collusion with any avoidance stemming from the PTSD and relationship problems.

We find that couples will complete assignments if there is expectation that they will do them and the therapist follows the principles just outlined. Realistically, couples do not routinely complete 100% of the OOSAs assigned. We aim for at least 75% adherence, yet we are consistently troubleshooting with the couple how they can further maximize their OOSAs. As we indicate in the session-by-session protocol that follows, if the couple comes to Session 4 and has not achieved at least 75% adherence, we strongly encourage the clinician and clients to revisit their treatment contract. Perhaps it is not the optimal time or circumstance to endeavor CBCT for PTSD. As a therapist, it is crucial to keep in mind the pitfalls of continuing with an evidence-based treatment protocol when your clients are minimally adherent. You run the risk of a partial response or nonresponse to treatment, which can leave the clients feeling hopeless, like a failure, and/or negative about evidence-based treatment. You or the next therapist also has that treatment history to overcome.

## Summary

CBCT for PTSD is built on a theoretical model that facilitates a dyadic conceptualization of posttraumatic mental health and relationship problems. It is time to move beyond individual-centric conceptions of posttraumatic stress problems to appreciate more fully the power of interpersonal relations in trauma recovery. Significant others play a critical role in engaging the traumatized individual in clinical services, maintaining their commitment to treatment, and promoting their recovery through therapy. This model is a time-limited and manualized therapy option for clinicians who might have minimal experience or confidence either in treating traumatized others or in providing a conjoint therapy to those who have been traumatized. The interventions making up CBCT for PTSD have empirical support in the individual PTSD and couple therapy outcome literatures. Moreover, the specific protocol has scientific and clinical evidence supporting its use in treating traumatic stress-related problems, enhancing the mental health and well-being of the significant others of those with these problems, and improving the relationship problems associated with these problems in order to live a quality life. We turn our attention next to assessment, case conceptualization, and therapy progress monitoring.

## CHAPTER 2

# Initial Assessment, Case Conceptualization, and Working with Complex Cases

Multiple emotional and behavioral problems are likely to arise after traumatic stress exposure (Kessler et al., 1995); consequently, a single diagnosis of PTSD is the exception rather than the rule. Moreover, and as noted earlier, research has consistently shown that the partners of those with PTSD often have their own mental health conditions, whether by virtue of living with someone with a mental health condition or because of their own individual mental health history. Thus, a comprehensive assessment of both the couple together and each person individually is required in the provision of quality care. Evidence-based assessment provides essential information for determining the appropriateness of the intervention for a given couple and for treatment planning.

## Who Is Appropriate for CBCT for PTSD?

Clinical interview and self-report assessment are important to determining whether a couple is a candidate for CBCT for PTSD and whether they are responding to the course of treatment. We recommend implementing the relatively liberal inclusion–exclusion criteria that we have used in clinical trials to determine whether couples are eligible for the intervention in clinical practice. At present, the intervention has been used with a range of traumatized individuals who vary with respect to type of index event, relationship satisfaction, and sexual orientation. Individual conditions or problems in either member of dyads whom we have excluded from treatment include (1) substance *dependence* (but we have included those with a substance *abuse* diagnosis), (2) *uncontrolled* severe mental health symptoms (i.e., active psychosis or mania; we have included those with this class of diagnosis if their symptoms were under relative control), (3) *severe* cognitive disorders, and (4) *imminent* suicidality and homicidality. We have emphasized particular words in these criteria because we have included individuals with substance abuse diagnoses, major mental health diagnoses that were stabilized, a history of traumatic brain injury and mild cognitive impairments, and those with active suicidality without intention to harm themselves. With regard to possible relationship-oriented exclusions, we exclude couples when one or both partners do not express at least *minimal* commitment to their relationship, which we have operationally defined as a willingness to commit to the 15 sessions of therapy with the intention of seeing whether the relationship can be improved. Ongoing infidelity is another exclusion criterion as is *severe* relationship aggression, which we have operationally defined consistent with the Revised Conflict Tactics Scales (CTS2; Straus, Hamby, Boney-McCoy, & Sugarman, 1996) and discuss later. We have fewer research data on couples in which both individuals are diagnosed with PTSD but are currently piloting the treatment.

## Recommended Assessment Process

We recommend three pretreatment sessions for assessment. If a couple is referred for the therapy, we recommend that you initially meet with them as a couple to hear their mutual rendition of couple-level problems, their expectations and hopes for the therapy, and their motivation for engaging in 15 sessions of couple therapy. To engender hopefulness for the couple, it is important to inquire about any times in the relationship when they experienced positive emotions and behaviors (e.g., when they started dating). In this first assessment session, the nature of the therapy (i.e., time limited, in- and out-of-session practice, trauma focused, systemic) should be explicitly discussed with the couple in order for them to provide fully informed consent to engage in the therapy. In addition to discussing the conventional limits of confidentiality in your specific jurisdiction, it is important in this session to establish the conjoint frame of the therapy by indicating that any information shared with the therapist without the other partner present *may* be shared by the therapist at his or her discretion in a couple session. This prevents you as the therapist from holding secrets and being held hostage by those secrets.

With the provision about sharing information in the couple context in place, the therapist is encouraged to schedule a second set of assessment sessions for each partner individually. At the second assessment meeting, the therapist takes one partner's history while the other completes brief objective measures of mental health and relationship difficulties (available at *www.coupletherapyforptsd.com*) in a quiet office area. When both are finished, the partners switch assessment assignments. We recommend a third assessment session in which the therapist provides feedback to the couple regarding individual and couple functioning, which reinforces the rationale for pursuing a course of CBCT for PTSD or for referral if PTSD or its symptoms are not relevant or there are reasons to exclude the couple from the therapy. In this approach, the fourth session with the couple would be the first session of the CBCT for PTSD protocol.

## Individual-Level Objective Assessment

### PTSD

In conducting the individual assessments, it is important for the therapist to establish whether either or both individuals meet diagnostic criteria for PTSD or have at least subthreshold levels.

A careful assessment of the traumatic event(s) informs diagnosis but also helps the therapist to anticipate the couple's likely avoidance issues and the nature of the trauma-focused cognitive work that will ensue in the third phase of the therapy. There are some traumas that may be particularly difficult to hear or discuss in a conjoint context given their extreme personal relevance to the partner. For example, a combatant's act of violence against a civilian may be very difficult to disclose to his or her partner. The guilt and shame associated with the act often leads the person to believe he or she is eternally and wholly bad and would be rejected by his or her partner upon disclosure. We recognize that these types of traumas may involve greater intensity of feeling and a more complex discussion for the couple but are not necessarily reasons to avoid a course of CBCT for PTSD.

If during individual assessment the PTSD+ partner discloses a trauma that is extremely personally relevant trauma for his or her partner, the therapist should discuss the potential costs and benefits of disclosing the general nature of the trauma to his or her partner in the context of CBCT for PTSD. Our stance is that partners should not usually be deterred from sharing these types of traumas within the therapy and with their partner so as to avoid inadvertently sending a message that what they did or did not do is unspeakable, horrific, or shameworthy. It is ultimately the client's decision as to whether he or she wants to pursue the therapy, with your clinical guidance about how the trauma can best be discussed in the conjoint context.

That said, we do not presume that CBCT for PTSD is a panacea; there may be some cases in which the therapy is not indicated because of the highly personally relevant content of the trauma for the partner (e.g., rape perpetration). However, we believe these cases to be relatively rare. We have had cases in which CBCT for PTSD was pursued with particularly personally relevant traumas for the partner (e.g., killing civilians in a war zone, sexual assault), and we provide examples of this work later within the protocol. A strength of CBCT for PTSD is that an explicit rendition of the trauma is not required in the trauma-focused phase in order for the therapy to work. It is also important to keep in mind that sometimes a partner's imagination about what happened or not knowing what happened is more problematic for the other partner than the knowledge of what actually happened.

A gold standard method of assessing the presence and severity of PTSD is the Clinician-Administered PTSD Scale (CAPS; Blake et al., 1995). The CAPS provides ratings for the frequency and severity of each of the DSM symptoms of PTSD, which can then be used to make a diagnosis of PTSD, and provides a quantitative measure of overall severity. In clinical practice, it may not be possible to conduct the CAPS to establish the *severity* of PTSD symptoms, in which case the PTSD Checklist (PCL; Weathers, Litz, Herman, Huska, & Keane, 1993) might be used as a substitute. The PCL is a brief (i.e., less than 5 minutes to complete) self-report measure that allows respondents to rate the severity of each of the PTSD symptoms. There is research suggesting that changes on the CAPS and PCL mirror each other over the course of treatment (Monson, Gradus, et al., 2008).

We have created and routinely use a partner version of the PCL, in which partners rate their perception of their loved one's PTSD symptoms. The partner's perception of the patient's PTSD symptoms can provide invaluable clinical information in general, especially in light of research and our own clinical experiences that some individuals with PTSD may not fully appreciate or may minimize or exaggerate their posttraumatic stress symptomatology. Discrepancies in the multimodal assessment of PTSD can provide important clinical information regarding case conceptualization and possible barriers to maximal treatment benefit.

## Other Conditions

It is important to assess for comorbid conditions, common among individuals with PTSD, such as major depression and substance use disorders. In addition, research indicates that the intimate partners of individuals with PTSD will likely present with their own mental health problems, with the symptoms of depression, substance abuse, and general anxiety being the most likely. This is, in part, why we encourage clinicians to meet with each partner individually and complete a structured interview, such as the Structured Clinical Interview for DSM-IV (First, Gibbon, Spitzer, & Williams, 1996) or Mini-International Neuropsychiatric Interview (M.I.N.I.; Sheehan et al., 1998), or have them complete at least a brief battery of self-report assessment instruments. Other brief, objective measures of these constructs that we recommend include the Beck Depression Inventory–II (Beck, Steer, & Brown, 1996) or other depression severity measure, substance misuse screening with the Alcohol Use Disorders Identification Test (Saunders, Aasland, Babor, & de la Fuente, 1993) and Drug Abuse Screening Test (Skinner, 1982), and the State–Trait Anxiety Inventory (Spielberger & Lushene, 1989) for general anxiety. Clinicians may want to administer other objective measures relevant to suspected conditions.

# Relationship-Level Objective Assessment

We recommend that each partner complete objective, self-report assessments of relationship satisfaction and intimate aggression as part of the initial assessment. Relationship satisfaction is not an inclusion–exclusion criterion for the therapy, although for the modal couple receiving CBCT for PTSD one or both partners has at least borderline relationship satisfaction. In our clinical settings and research protocols, we treat couples who have engaged in minor acts of aggression according to objective assessment and include cessation of physical aggression as a treatment goal. We provide referrals for individual or group treatment for clients or couples who are engaging in more severe forms of aggression.

## Relationship Adjustment

The Dyadic Adjustment Scale (DAS; Spanier, 1976) is the most frequently used measure of intimate relationship satisfaction or adjustment. The DAS has been shown to discriminate between distressed and nondistressed couples and to correctly identify couples with a high likelihood of divorce (e.g., Crane, Busby, & Larson, 1991). A clinical cutoff total score of 98 or less has been shown to be an efficient indicator for relationship satisfaction. In addition, a single item on the DAS regarding overall relationship happiness accounts for approximately 80% of the variance in relationship satisfaction (Sharpley & Cross, 1982), and we use this item across sessions to gauge changes in satisfaction.

## Intimate Aggression

When working with distressed couples, it is essential to assess for aggression and violence, because research indicates that at least 50% of presenting couples report a history of physical aggression in their relationship in the past year (e.g., O'Leary & Williams, 2006; Sherman,

Sautter, Jackson, Lyons, & Xiaotong, 2006). Assessing for aggression and violence is especially important when at least one member of the dyad has PTSD. The hyperarousal symptoms of PTSD, such as sleep disturbance, irritability/anger, difficulty concentrating, hypervigilance, and an exaggerated startle response, have been found to be associated with intimate aggression perpetration (Savarese, Suvak, King, & King, 2001). Furthermore, male and female war veterans diagnosed with PTSD, compared with those without PTSD, are more likely to perpetrate verbal and physical aggression against their partners and children (Carroll et al., 1985; Glenn et al., 2002; Gold et al., 2007; Jordan et al., 1992; Verbosky & Ryan, 1988), with rates as high as 63% for some act of physical violence in the past year (Byrne & Riggs, 1996).

The most widely used and well-supported measure to assess for couple aggression is the CTS2 (Straus et al., 1996). This 78-item self-report measure is completed by both partners and is used to assess three modes of conflict resolution: positive conflict behavior, psychological aggression, and physical assault. The CTS2 is behaviorally anchored and yields three subscales that coincide with the three modes of conflict resolution. Furthermore, the scale includes items to assess sexual coercion/assault and physical injury. Because both partners complete the measure independently, the clinician gains useful information about concordance between partners' responses.

Important to note in the assessment of intimate violence is that precautions should be taken to minimize any risk to partners that might come with reporting aggression (e.g., measures should be completed independently and privately). Moreover, the objective assessment of violence should be followed up with questions about perceived safety if experiences of aggression are reported. These questions should be asked in private meetings, and the clinician should be careful to explore any concerns about sharing the report of aggression experiences with the other partner. Safety planning may be necessary; this is yet another reason for individual meetings with partners.

## *Communication*

Assessing a couple's communication patterns yields important information about the strengths and problematic communication behaviors to be targeted in the treatment. This information is clinically useful and informs case conceptualization and treatment planning. We encourage you, as the clinician, to collect a behavioral sample just before the first session of therapy, during which you ask the couple to communicate for 5 to 10 minutes about a moderately distressing issue in their relationship while you observe. Collecting the communication sample just before the first session of the protocol allows you to easily segue into the content of the first session, which includes sharing that a major intervention in the treatment is improved communication.

### *Setup*

The setup for the communication sample should be relatively brief. The "three R's" of setting up the communication sample include:

1. *Rationale for the sample.* A major aspect of the treatment involves improving the couple's communication. Thus, you want to get a window into their current strengths and difficulties in communicating with one another to provide targeted treatment.
2. *Representative sample.* You want the couple to communicate as similarly as possible to

how they communicate at home. Your job is to be as nonintrusive as possible in listening and watching. However, it is important to normalize that they might feel awkward, at least initially, as you are there observing their communication.
3. *Right size of topic.* You want to have the couple choose a topic that is *moderately distressing* in their relationship (how they negotiate this choice is also important information to collect). If the topic is too "hot" or too "cold," you are not as likely to get a good sense of their communication skills. Examples of typical topics include finances, division of household chores, parenting, in-laws, and family–work balance.

A sample of the introduction follows:

*As I mentioned in our assessment session, one of the major parts of the treatment is improving your communication. Before we start, I would like to get a window into the way that you currently communicate with one another.*

*I'd like you to communicate with one another as closely as possible to how you communicate at home. That will give me the best information about things you seem to be doing well and other things that we can work on to improve your relationship. I will be here in the room, but I'm going to ask you to turn your chairs toward each other, and I will move my chair back and stay out of your way as much as possible while you are talking. It might feel awkward, at least at first, but I'd like you to try to communicate as closely as possible to how you communicate at home.*

*Choose a topic that is moderately distressing for the two of you to talk about—not your greatest source of conflict and not something minor that you barely disagree about either. It is okay if your conversation moves on to other topics, but we will start with this topic. Can the two of you think of something that is moderately distressing to talk about?*

It is not necessary that the partners choose the "right" topic to discuss. Couples will tend to discuss the important topics, no matter where they start, and their typical manner of communicating will be displayed. Allow the partners to communicate between 5 and 10 minutes.

## What to Look for in Communication Samples

Here are a few things to look for in the communication sample:

*Strengths to Highlight*
- Do they naturally paraphrase or clarify?
- Is there eye contact?
- Do they share emotions? Is there a range of emotions shared?
- Is there a balance in the amount of time each person spends communicating?

*Concerns to Address*
- Is there hostility, contemptuousness, or disgust conveyed via vocal tone or nonverbals (e.g., eye rolling, heavy sighing)?
- Is there any name calling?

- Is there exaggerated language (e.g., "always," "never," "all the time")?
- Is there mind reading?
- What does their body language convey (e.g., openness, defensiveness, indifference, closeness)
- Do they interrupt each other?

## Feedback

When you end the sample period, be sure to thank the couple for giving you the opportunity to observe their communication and tell them how helpful it will be to you in planning their treatment. Also, it is helpful to ask them how representative the conversation was relative to conversations they have at home ("On a scale of 1–10, with 10 being exactly similar, how similar was this conversation to those you have at home on these topics?").

Then be sure to point out *at least* one strength that you observed to instill hope for change. Even for the most distressed couples, you can always say that they are at least still talking with one another. Also, indicate that you believe you can help them to improve the way they communicate with one another and thereby improve their relationship.

You can then transition into the content of the first session of the therapy, reminding the couple that improving their communication is one of the key targets of the therapy.

# How Assessment Guides Therapy: Case Conceptualization in CBCT for PTSD

After the assessment information has been gathered, the therapist has the important task of fitting the pieces of information together for the purposes of case conceptualization. In conceptualizing cases, we consider how individual- and relationship-level variables interact to maintain PTSD and associated relationship difficulties and illustrate this process using a case example, as follows.

> Susan and Jake presented for couple therapy as a result of difficulties with communication and intimacy that a previous therapist suspected might be at least partly due to Susan's experience of having been raped while in college. Both were in their mid-30s and had been romantically involved for 5 years, living together for 3 of them. During the first meeting with the therapist, the couple reported that they cared deeply for each other but felt as if something was always "between" them despite their best efforts to bridge that gap. They described feeling happy, almost euphoric, in the early months of their relationship, but that, as things became more serious, problems developed and persisted. Susan stated that she loved Jake but felt as though she could not help becoming very angry at him at times for seemingly no reason. Jake described, in turn, how Susan frequently accused him of trying to control her and provided a recent example: A week earlier Jake offered to drive since Susan seemed tired, but she interpreted this as Jake thinking she was a bad driver and that he was trying to make her feel like a child. Jake also described Susan's jumpiness when he tried to touch her physically in any way, including holding her hand or giving her a hug. Susan replied, "Well, when you do things like that and I don't expect it, I assume that you're trying to

hurt me!" Sexual contact had become practically nonexistent at the point at which they presented for therapy. Attempts to discuss this and other topics usually started out in the form of bickering but escalated, ending with one or both of them shouting. Jake stated that to avoid frightening Susan or provoking her anger, he pulled back and tried to be extremely careful around her, to the point of feeling as though he were "walking on eggshells." Jake added that he had recently found multiple empty bottles of wine and had observed Susan to be withdrawn, suspecting that she was probably drinking more than she should. Susan hotly denied this and pointed to this as further proof that he was trying to control her. Jake said that he felt sad a lot of the time and was discouraged about the state of their relationship. At the time that they presented for treatment, the couple had not had sex in nearly 2 years, rarely went out on dates, and reported feeling as though they were living like "roommates" instead of as a couple. Nonetheless, they both said that they were committed to each other and wanted to do whatever they could to improve their relationship.

After meeting with each partner and reviewing their self-report measures, the therapist began to formulate the couple's case. She determined that Susan met criteria for current PTSD, chronic major depressive disorder, and recurrent, moderate alcohol abuse; and that Jake met criteria for current dysthymic disorder and past marijuana dependence, in sustained full remission. Susan's responses on the PCL placed her in the severe range of symptom severity, whereas Jake's ratings placed her in the mild to moderate range. The therapist conceptualized Susan's drinking behavior as an avoidance strategy to manage her distress and her depression as a result of feeling chronically helpless to manage her own emotions and the effect of this on her relationship. Jake's low mood was understood as resulting from his feeling chronically distressed about their relationship but unable to improve the situation. At the relationship level, their responses on the DAS revealed Susan to be in the low satisfied range and Jake to be in the clinically distressed range. On the CTS2, both denied ever striking one another but did endorse several instances of name calling and throwing of objects within the previous year.

The therapist determined that, in addition to the presence of relationship distress, the couple was accommodating Susan's symptoms. Jake's efforts to avoid situations that might provoke Susan's anxiety or anger and their couple-level avoidance of physical intimacy and going out to public places were actually maintaining both Susan's symptoms and their relationship problems, because the couple had learned to adopt a general strategy of avoiding rather than approaching uncomfortable situations. This reinforced Susan's belief that the world was an unsafe place and interfered with both emotional and physical intimacy. The therapist also suspected that the discrepancy between their perceptions of the severity of Susan's PTSD symptoms further contributed to distress on Jake's part, because he saw Susan's behavior toward him as a lack of caring rather than as a reflection of the severity of her symptoms. The therapist hypothesized that psychoeducation about PTSD and its effects on relationships would help to address this. In addition, the therapist also anticipated having more information about the couple's interacting trauma-relevant cognitions after they completed the TIQs as OOSAs after Session 1. She would then have information about how each made sense of or appraised Susan's sexual trauma and their beliefs across trauma- and interpersonally relevant areas. She would be better equipped to understand how their respective cognitions might interact to maintain posttraumatic stress symptoms and relationship distress and thus to intervene effectively.

With regard to emotional functioning, Susan was struggling with anger and fear dysregulation. The therapist suspected that Susan was likely experiencing guilt and shame related to the sexual assault, because of a comment during her individual clinical interview that she wished she hadn't been drinking at the time of the assault. Jake's low mood seemed to influence his perception of Susan, and Susan tended to make negative, self-critical attributions about Jake's mood, further exacerbating her own negative emotions. Their negative and reciprocally exchanged emotions had contributed to the deterioration of their relationship intimacy and overall satisfaction, which, in turn, was contributing to individual stress and the clinical symptom picture.

Having determined that a course of CBCT for PTSD was appropriate and indicated, the therapist met with the couple for a third session to provide feedback from the assessment and to explain of how treatment would target Susan's PTSD symptoms and their relationship problems, with the expectation that Susan's alcohol use problems and each partner's mood difficulties would improve as well.

## How Do We Know They're Getting Better?: Ongoing Assessment

Over the course of therapy, we recommend that both partners complete the respective versions of the PCL at the beginning of each session, reporting on symptoms over the past week. We also recommend that some brief assessment of relationship satisfaction be administered to evaluate ongoing functioning (as mentioned, we use the single overall happiness item from the DAS). Because of their brevity, we recommend that these across-treatment sessions be done every other session if treatment is delivered twice per week. If treatment is delivered once per week, then we recommend that the assessments be done every session (see session-by-session protocol in Part II). Other relevant (comorbid) conditions in the partners should also be monitored. This assessment information should be conveyed to the couple to reinforce progress or to determine impediments to a successful course of therapy.

## Working with Complex Cases

We recognize that not all cases are created equal and that there are certain clinical issues whose management merits special attention in order to deliver the protocol effectively. Working with couples with comorbidities and complex presentations is more challenging for the therapist. However, we have successfully treated the majority of these cases in treatment outcome studies and in clinical practice outside the context of research (e.g., Monson et al., 2011). It is also important to mention that we have been humbled over time about our ability to predict which couples will profit from CBCT for PTSD. Our own personal humbling is consistent with the literature on the prediction of PTSD outcomes (i.e., there are relatively few consistent predictors of treatment outcomes in PTSD; e.g., van Minnen, Arntz, & Keijsers, 2002). We mention this because clinicians can have preconceived notions about the types of couples or individuals who will respond best to the treatment (e.g., young, affluent, high intellect, less trauma history). These ideas can serve as self-fulfilling prophecies for the therapist and couple. We assert that everyone deserves a fair shot at empirically supported therapy and stand by the most consistently observed research finding in the CBT literature: that out-of-session practice is the single best predictor of treatment outcomes (Kazantzis et al., 2000). In other words, what the couple puts into the therapy, they will get out of it.

For the purposes of this discussion, we group these considerations in treating more complex cases according to whether they are individual comorbidities or relationship comorbidities. In addition to the comorbidity factors, we offer some specific guidance and recommendations to help you deliver CBCT for PTSD to a range of couples, presented next.

## Individual Comorbidities

### Problematic Substance Use

Although a substance *dependence* diagnosis for either partner is currently an exclusion criterion for this treatment, a substance *abuse* diagnosis is not. Nonetheless, maladaptive substance use still needs to be addressed because of its potential to compromise the treatment's potency. As previously discussed, we consider substance misuse to serve as a form of emotional avoidance. That is, drinking alcohol, smoking marijuana, and/or using other drugs to cope with trauma-related cues deprives the traumatized individual of the opportunity to experience uncomfortable emotions or other sensations in the context of feared situations but then learn a sense of safety when he or she is, in fact, safe. From a cognitive perspective, using substances in the face of distress also reinforces the belief that the only way to manage one's discomfort is to escape or avoid it.

When working with couples in which one or both partners misuse substances, we recommend first getting their buy-in to the conceptualization of substance use as a form of avoidance that maintains the disorder and relationship problems, much like behavioral avoidance of feared situations, and then contracting for decreased use. You will note that we do not necessarily require abstinence as a treatment goal but rather moderated use across contexts as well as refraining from use before sessions or when doing out-of-session practice assignments. For patients who are reluctant to curb their use, we have found it useful to frame decreased use as an experiment to see what happens to their mental health symptoms and their relationship functioning when they are not using or are using less. At the dyadic level, and in keeping with the systemic nature of CBCT for PTSD, it is important to address the symptom–system fit problem that we have previously mentioned (i.e., ways that the couple may have evolved their relationship to inadvertently maintain symptom expression; Rohrbaugh et al., 1985) by helping them generate alternative couple activities if drinking is a shared activity and by addressing any partner tendencies to encourage the patient's drinking or other substance use as a way of managing distress.

We consider lapses in use to be part of the learning process and not necessarily an indication that the substance-misusing individuals cannot change or that therapy should be discontinued. After all, he or she has learned to use substances to cope with distress, and substance use is powerfully and negatively reinforced because it is connected with the removal of an unpleasant state. Change rarely happens overnight. Therefore, in the event of a lapse to substance misuse, it is important to normalize it, determine the contextual factors at play that might have contributed to it, and treat it as important information for how they, as a couple, can respond differently with increased skill use. When working with couples, we have also found this topic to be an excellent opportunity to practice the communications skills introduced in Phase 2 of the therapy, particularly when there are differences of opinion between partners about what constitutes appropriate use. Couples can use their sharing thoughts and feelings skills to clarify each person's needs and wants around the issue (e.g., what do they each feel comfortable with in terms of use and why is this important to them?) and can then transition to using their problem-solving skills to decide how to proceed in situations in which alcohol or drugs might be present and what they, as a couple, will do if either or both appear to be vulnerable to using more or have used more than agreed upon. The interpersonally oriented cognitive strategy introduced in Session 6 can also be useful in challenging either partner's black-and-white thinking that one lapse is tantamount to failure or confirmation that things can never get better.

## Dissociation

Research suggests that dissociation shares similar biological and psychological underpinnings with emotional numbing and serves a function similar to other avoidant behaviors (Frewen & Lanius, 2006). Although dissociation may initially be an automatic freeze-oriented response when feeling helpless in the face of a perceived life-threatening situation, over time it can become an overlearned response to any form of distress. The dissociative behavior is connected with the temporary removal of an aversive state. As with substance misuse, this extreme form of experiential avoidance interferes with new learning because the individual is deprived of the opportunity to tolerate uncomfortable emotions in the context of feared situations and to learn how to discern accurately between being in danger versus being safe. Similarly, it also reinforces the belief that the individual cannot endure an anxiety-provoking situation without mentally "checking out."

We have found that it is possible to address dissociation effectively in the context of CBCT for PTSD because many of the interventions serve to disrupt dissociative processes. We have had success with several strategies, all of which focus on helping the dissociative individual remain in the here and now. For example, the therapist is encouraged to send smaller portions of information when speaking and to ask the patient to paraphrase what he or she received during the session to decrease the likelihood that he or she will dissociate. As early as possible in treatment, we advise having the patient and partner take active roles in managing dissociation by their becoming increasingly skilled at recognizing early warning signs of dissociation (e.g., the patient is staring off or not paying attention) as well as possible triggers for the dissociation (e.g., feeling physically warm or anxious). Having the partner check in with the patient regarding the material he or she took in during the session and helping to physically ground the patient by holding hands or placing a hand on the patient's shoulder if that would be comfortable to the patient once he or she indicates that dissociation has occurred can further increase the probability of the patient remaining present during the session. Couples are encouraged to use these same skills outside of session to combat dissociation and increase emotional tolerance and regulation. In addition, and starting in Session 3, having the partners use paraphrasing skills and speaking in short talk turns can also serve to increase the patient's engagement in the conversation and tolerance for distressing topics.

## Severe Depression

Severe depression is not an exclusion criterion for CBCT for PTSD, except when the patient is *imminently* suicidal. These circumstances notwithstanding, individuals with severe depression can still benefit from treatment, although the therapist should be mindful of ways that the mood disturbance may complicate treatment. For instance, we have seen a number of cases in which one partner suffered from severe major depression and experienced chronic passive suicidality as a result of feelings of extreme hopelessness. Because suicidal ideation can be anxiety provoking for the clinician, patient, and partner, there can be an understandable pull to spend most of the session(s) discussing the suicidal ideation, even though an evaluation indicates that the patient is not at imminent risk of self-harm. As a consequence, the causes of the suicidal ideation might not get addressed as the primary problem. Even when suicidal ideation is not a salient feature of the presenting problem, complications can arise when depressed individuals do not exert as much effort as needed to fully complete their OOSAs because of depressive beliefs that the skills will not work anyway, so why try. Severe depression can also complicate OOSA completion because of difficulties with behavioral activation, when the individual finds it hard to mobilize the energy needed to do the exercises as assigned.

We find it helpful to externalize depressive thinking patterns and behaviors by framing the traumatic experience(s) as the cause of these patterns and behaviors and an external influence on the couple's relationship that must be collaboratively fought against by both partners. In addition, we conceptualize suicidal thinking as escape behavior in the face of hopelessness and frame the hopelessness itself as a thought that things cannot get better. These thoughts can then be explored with the dyadic cognitive strategy described in Chapter 1. For patients who say things like, "I didn't do the assignment because there's no point, and I just don't believe that it's going to work," we recommend trying to capitalize on their unwillingness to believe something without evidence to the contrary through therapist responses such as, "I see that you bring some healthy skepticism to the table, which is great because we're actually going to use that to our advantage during treatment." In this spirit, it is often useful to engage the couple in treating the early OOSAs focused on behavioral skill use as an experiment through statements such as, "Let's see what happens to the symptoms and your relationship as you both give it your all with these assignments." Often, once the couple starts doing the Phase 1 exercises designed to increase positivity and decrease conflict, negative thoughts about themselves, their partners, and the world more generally start to shift. You can also leverage the patient's desire for hard evidence as a prerequisite for changing his or her mind when you introduce the cognitive strategy in Session 6: "I see that you want evidence or proof before you're willing to believe something. Let's put that healthy skepticism to good use by examining thoughts that each of you have that are maintaining the PTSD and relationship difficulties and see how you feel once we start to consider multiple ways of looking at things." Such therapist statements can help to avoid power struggles with depressed individuals who insist on maintaining certain beliefs and gently introduce the notion that there can be more than one way of viewing a situation.

To reinforce these efforts on a behavioral level and in keeping with principles of behavioral activation for depression, we recommend programming *in vivo* approach activities that double as shared rewarding activities for the relationship but also provide a sense of mastery and pleasure for the depressed individual(s) starting in Session 4. Although there is wide variability across patients and partners in terms of what activities promote mastery or pleasure, exercise or other activities that involve physical activity are likely good places to start.

## *Personality Disorders*

The affective dysregulation and cognitive rigidity that characterize certain personality disorders (e.g., Cluster B personality disorders) can interact with emotion regulation difficulties and maladaptive thinking patterns common to the disorders that most commonly occur after traumatic stress exposure. Furthermore, in the context of a highly discordant relationship, personality disorder symptoms can contribute to significant emotional and behavioral volatility and further increase risk for verbal and physical aggression.

In the absence of current or imminent self-harm behaviors at the individual level or severe physical aggression at the dyadic level, we believe that couples in which one or both partners have a personality disorder or personality disorder features can be treated successfully, provided that the therapist is able and willing to contain the couple when needed, to be explicit about expectations and contingencies for treatment, and to enforce these as indicated. To manage affect dysregulation in one or both partners, it is often necessary to implement a higher degree of structure. In this vein, we recommend that the therapist strongly encourage and reinforce skill use in and out of sessions, closely containing any emotionally aggressive behavior between partners or toward the therapist. High levels of dysregulation during sessions also require more active and direct intervention on the part of the therapist, and it is essential for the therapist to firmly redirect couples if they engage in high levels of conflict. The therapist's swift intervention—by calling a time-out and shortening talk turns—is crucial and also serves as an important way to model skill use for couples who have difficulty engaging such skills in the midst of intense emotions. For couples who balk at being directed in this manner, it is helpful to highlight that such relationship interactions serve to maintain traumatic stress-related problems by reinforcing the idea that the traumatized person is still under threat, which, in turn, interferes with recovery. We have also found it useful to remind them gently, in a nonconfrontational manner, that they have sought out your services in order to learn a different way of relating, and that you believe that you would not be doing your job if you permitted them to reenact problematic relationship behaviors during the session.

In general, we advise having as little between-session contact with clients as possible in order to encourage the couple's self-reliance and distress tolerance and to discourage potential triangulation with the therapist, especially in the event that one partner calls with the intention of trying to "get you on their side." If one or both members of the couple contact you outside of session in a crisis, you should inquire about skills they have already used to manage their distress and then coach them in thinking through which skills they can use to communicate better between now and their next session.

There may be instances in which one or both partners' maladaptive behaviors are unwittingly reinforced and thereby interfere with recovery from trauma and maintain relationship problems. It is important to watch for this and other ways in which these maladaptive relationship interactions are maintained and to discuss the consequences. For example, a patient with borderline personality disorder features predicted that she would emotionally "fall apart" and would need to self-harm if her partner did not do what she wanted. To avoid provoking the patient's distress, the partner acquiesced to her wishes but, in so doing, felt emotionally distressed himself as a result of feeling "held hostage." In cases such as this, it is important for the therapist to highlight that this interactional pattern actually serves to maintain the patient's problems because it reinforces the patient's belief that he or she could not tolerate his or her own emotions and serves to maintain relationship distress because the partner is not getting his or her own needs met. We have also found it helpful to discuss potential implications for treatment if the dysregulated behaviors persist. For example, if the patient is so dysregulated that treatment cannot proceed as prescribed, he or she may need to be referred for a higher level of care that specifically targets these maladaptive behaviors, such as dialectical behavior therapy (Linehan, 1993). The intention is to return to CBCT for PTSD when there is better affective and behavioral control. As noted previously in the context of severe depression, we recommend addressing cognitive rigidity in the context of personality disorders by labeling the thoughts as hypotheses that can be tested in the face of skill use.

## *Relationship Comorbidities*

### *Physical Aggression*

As noted earlier, physical aggression is a commonly co-occurring problem among couples who present for couple therapy, even though most do not seek help with intimate aggression per se. In the context of PTSD, the risk of physical aggression is increased because of hyperarousal symptoms and may be further amplified in the presence of substance use. In the course of our work, we have seen couples from a wide range of socioeconomic statuses, cultural backgrounds, and sexual orientations engage in some form of physical aggression, even though the presenting problem was one partner's PTSD symptoms. We have also found that, in the case of mild physical aggression (e.g., pushing, throwing objects), the aggression is often bidirectional. Therefore, it is imperative to inquire about the presence of physical aggression for all couples who present for treatment in order to ensure that conjoint therapy is appropriate and, if there is aggression, to enhance treatment planning by including the elimination of physical aggression by both partners as an explicit treatment goal.

To be able to do the hard work of treatment, especially a trauma-focused one such as CBCT for PTSD, physical safety is a prerequisite for emotional safety. This is essential because if the environment is not physically safe, the traumatized partner cannot view him- or herself as having been in danger in the past but safe in the here and the now. The sense of current safety needed for recovery from PTSD also extends to emotional safety because, to the extent that the traumatized individual is in a physically or emotionally threatening environment, he or she will continue to view him- or herself as under threat, and PTSD and relationship problems will be maintained. In the case of aggression perpetrated by the partner with PTSD, we have also found that the aggression can serve a functional role in maintaining PTSD-related avoidance and problems with emotional intimacy (e.g., "If I am verbally or physically aggressive toward you, then I don't have to risk being close to you").

As discussed in the prior chapter on assessment, it is important to assess partners separately about physical aggression to decrease the risk of acquiescent responding and to develop a safety plan in the event that one or both partners feels unsafe. Couples engaging in severe physical or sexual aggression are not appropriate candidates for couple treatment while the aggression is ongoing and need to be referred for individual treatment focused on the aggressive behavior until it is better managed. If the couple is motivated for treatment but conjoint therapy is contraindicated at the present time, one option available to the clinician is to institute a trial period while one or both partners are in individual therapy to determine whether they, as a couple, can refrain from aggression as a condition to undertake a course of conjoint treatment at a later time.

For couples engaging in more minor forms of physical or sexual aggression, we strongly recommend setting the elimination of all aggression as a treatment goal in the first session and having both partners sign the contract committing to this. Because verbal aggression (e.g., yelling, name calling, other forms of hostility) can be a harbinger of physical aggression, we also advise that clinicians and couples include the elimination of verbal aggression as an explicit treatment goal at the end of Session 1. We introduce conflict management skills early in treatment (i.e., in the second session of Phase 1) to provide couples with the important foundation of physical and emotional safety so that they can maximally profit from the couple-level behavioral and cognitive interventions used in Phases 2 and 3. In addition, we make sure that they practice the interventions during the session to increase the likelihood of their practicing them out of session. This includes noticing the early warning signs of anger, practicing slowed breathing, and, perhaps most importantly, using time-out. In the event that couples cannot refrain from engaging in aggressive acts or if aggression escalates during treatment, you should have an immediate discussion with them about the challenge of continuing with the protocol given that it is difficult, if not impossible, to recover from past traumas if the current environment is not physically safe. If the couple continues to engage in physical aggression, you should consider stopping the protocol and discussing referrals for individual therapy focused on the physically aggressive behavior.

## Ambivalence about Being in the Relationship

By the time couples seek treatment for relationship distress, it is not uncommon that one or both partners have strongly considered ending the relationship and feel ambivalent about continuing it. For some couples, this ambivalence may be shared during a mutually honest, respectful conversation in which they both agree that things are not working and that it might be best to end the relationship. However, for many, the frustration, resentment, and sense of despair that characterize chronically distressed relationships can contribute to ongoing threats to leave the relationship, especially during times of acute conflict. Although understandable, this type of behavior is extremely corrosive to a relationship and causes destabilization because it undermines a sense of safety, trust, and togetherness in working through what are typically co-created problems.

Many times, this ambivalence is driven by the thought, "Things have been bad for so long, how can they possibly get better?" It is helpful to normalize this sentiment and to introduce the notion that it is not that the relationship is doomed, but rather that trauma-related problems have been "pushing them around." Helping couples understand that hyperarousal symptoms contribute to poor conflict management skills and that avoidance and emotional numbing symptoms contribute to problems feeling close to one another can help to externalize the problems and increase a sense of hopefulness that perhaps the problems are due to the presence of a third party in their relationship—that is, PTSD—as opposed to an inherent problem in the relationship per se. Much in the way we address hopelessness in the context of depression, we encourage ambivalent couples to refrain from threats to leave the relationship during the course of treatment and to find alternative ways to express their relational distress with each other. We also encourage them to observe what happens when each puts his or her best foot forward and does the exercises as intended. Many times, the outlook on the relationship and its possibilities becomes more positive as couples think and behave differently toward each other, with resulting changes in how they feel about each other. In some cases, couples might still ultimately decide to end their relationship after completing a full course of therapy, but at least they can know they gave it their best efforts and can feel good about the thoughtful process they engaged in to come to this decision as opposed to acting impulsively.

## Infidelity

Ongoing infidelity in a relationship that is believed to be monogamous, whether sexual or emotional in nature, is a contraindication for this intervention and for couple therapy more generally. Infidelity is incompatible with a commitment to working on the relationship and contributes to one or both partners feeling emotionally unsafe in the relationship; it also interferes with the ability to establish and maintain trust. Furthermore, in cases when a traumatized partner is the one participating in the affair, it can reinforce trauma-related beliefs that the only reason someone would want to be involved with him or her is another's self-gratification and that it is impossible to have a relationship characterized by mutual emotional vulnerability and intimacy. Conversely, if the partner is the one having the affair, it can reinforce the patient's trauma-related beliefs that no one can be trusted.

Consistent with Baucom, Snyder, and Gordon's (2009) model of infidelity and its treatment, following the discovery of infidelity in a relationship presumed to be monogamous, many individuals will be in an acute state of emotional distress as they struggle to reconcile the affair with their previously held beliefs about themselves, their partner, and their relationship, and the couple will need a period of stabilization before they can do the difficult work of comprehending the infidelity and deciding how to move forward. Needless to say, this state of crisis can impede the couple's ability to participate successfully in a course of trauma-focused therapy because such work requires a sense of both individual- and couple-level stability. There is wide variability in the time it takes couples to achieve an adequate level of stabilization; therefore, clinicians will need to use their own judgment to determine whether this has occurred. For guidance on how to assist couples with this process, we recommend Baucom and colleagues' (2009) *Helping Couples Get Past the Affair*.

With stabilization, we encourage clinicians to conceptualize infidelity as a relationship comorbidity that may be related to the presence of PTSD and/or contribute to relationship distress. A history of infidelity is not an exclusion criterion for CBCT for PTSD. In the course of the assessment, you might determine that PTSD symptoms functionally contributed to the patient's participating in the affair as a way of avoiding intimacy with the partner or of managing distressing emotions more generally (e.g., "If I am not exclusively involved, then I don't have to risk being close to or emotionally intimate with [my partner]" or "If I am focused on the excitement of having sex with another person, I can distract myself from thinking about the trauma"). Similarly, if the partner engages in an affair, it can be important to consider and address how this has amplified the patient's PTSD symptoms in light of difficulties with trust that already existed or how difficulties with intimacy contributed to the affair behavior. If both partners are willing to focus treatment on their relationship vis-à-vis the PTSD specifically, then it is appropriate to conduct a course of CBCT for PTSD with them. On the other hand, if the participating partner is unwilling to stop the affair and/or one or both partners are so distressed that they want the focus of treatment to be on stabilization, then CBCT for PTSD is contraindicated. In this case, a reasonable next step is to make a referral for individual therapy or couple therapy focused on the causes and consequences of the infidelity so that they can move past the affair regardless of whether or not they decide to stay together as a couple.

As when discussing the patient's trauma, we strongly discourage discussing the affair in nitty-gritty detail, even though some partners may want to know exactly what sexual acts were performed, as well as when and where, as a way of helping them make sense of why the affair happened. Instead, it is more constructive for the discussion to remain at the level of broad brush strokes (e.g., "The affair was with a colleague during this period but is now over"). As with the trauma-focused portion of treatment in Phase 3, we recommend preparing the couple for the eventual goal of addressing maladaptive cognitions about the affair by considering the historical and proximate contexts that contributed to its occurrence, without necessarily condoning its having occurred in the first place. When one partner has trauma-related problems and it is determined that their symptoms are functionally related to the occurrence of the affair, treatment might involve a discussion of how stress in the relationship contributed to an increase in symptoms and that the patient felt that the only way to avoid thinking about the disturbing memories was to distract through sex with another person who showered them with attention and affection.

## Alternative Applications and Coordination with Other Interventions

CBCT for PTSD was originally designed to be delivered to individual intimate couples as a stand-alone treatment for PTSD and the enhancement of intimate relationship functioning, and we have the most empirical evidence to support its use in this format. However, we have clinical experience and uncontrolled data supporting the intervention's efficacy when delivered in multicouple groups, in individual and group formats with nonromantic dyads (e.g., parent–son, close friends), and with individuals whose significant others were unwilling or unable to participate in the therapy. We also recommend delivering phases of the intervention in tandem with individual trauma-focused interventions if the entire CBCT for PTSD protocol is not going to be used. We begin with a presentation of alternative applications of CBCT for PTSD and conclude with a discussion of issues to consider when using phases of the treatment in concert with individual evidence-based treatment.

### *Nonintimate Dyads*

In developing the protocol, we purposefully labeled the intervention a "conjoint" versus "couple" intervention because we envisioned its use beyond romantic couples to include a range of dyads composed of close others. In fact, it is our experience that nonromantic dyads presenting for treatment share more similarities than differences compared with romantic dyads. The typical nonromantic close other willing to participate in the treatment is someone who is quite invested in the health and well-being of the patient (e.g., family member, close friend) and likely affected by the traumatic stress symptoms.

Several differences that may arise in the delivery of the intervention with nonromantic dyads include completion of the OOSAs when the dyad does not live together and the coverage of physical intimacy in Session 13. With regard to the former, we suggest that the dyad and therapist troubleshoot how they will complete the OOSAs while living apart. For example, they may need to practice the communication skills over the phone, by e-mail, or through web-based videoconferencing (with appropriate caution regarding privacy). In these cases, we have also found it helpful for each member of the dyad to have a copy of the OOSAs so that they both have the relevant materials to reference and record responses. It is important to note that we have treated romantic couples who are not cohabitating, and these strategies also apply to them.

People often equate the topic of physical intimacy with sexual contact. As discussed in the protocol, we conceptualize physical closeness as a broader concept, with sexual contact as but one form of it. Physical closeness encompasses a range of circumstances, from physical proximity to strangers or acquaintances (e.g., on public transportation or in a public place) to the affectionate touch of loved ones, such as children, family members, friends, and intimate partners. There are some types of nonromantic dyads in which discussion of thoughts about sexual intimacy might be inappropriate (e.g., parent–child dyad), and in those cases we suggest that the therapist initiate a straightforward discussion about the parameters of the material that the dyad will discuss and encourage the patient to use cognitive strategies on any cognitions that he or she might not feel comfortable sharing with the loved one who is participating in the therapy.

## *Dual-PTSD Couples*

In couples in which both partners suffer from PTSD, the patterns and problems that arise are similar to those we have seen in many other couples treated with the protocol but tend to be amplified because of the traumatic stress-related psychopathology of both partners. Many of the couples we have treated were dyads in which both partners had trauma histories, which is not surprising given the relatively high rates of traumatic stress exposure documented in epidemiological studies. Fewer couples in which both partners meet criteria for a PTSD diagnosis have presented for therapy, but these dual-PTSD couples account for still a sizable minority. Thus, we have begun to test the therapy with these couples in a series of case studies and have treated them in clinical practice. We offer some suggestions based on our experience to date.

Consistent with the more detailed discussion of comorbidities and clinical complexities presented earlier in this chapter, these couples generally have more relationship distress and relationship comorbidities (e.g., aggression, infidelity) to manage in session and to address for successful completion of OOSAs. Consequently, the therapist typically needs to be more active and directive to contain the couple's interactions in the therapy sessions. However, we have also seen cases in which avoidance was predominant, and the partners were mutually disengaged as a means of decreasing affective experience and expression, which, in turn, decreased their intimacy and satisfaction. In this situation, the therapist's goal is to encourage expression of a range of affect, increase tolerance of affect in the relationship, and challenge thoughts that might interfere with emotional sharing (e.g., "If we share negative emotions, it will inevitably destroy our relationship").

In addition to the therapy process suggestions offered previously, there are some practical considerations regarding delivery of the protocol interventions to dual-PTSD couples. First, the therapist should be sure that the psychoeducation is relevant to both members of the couple and that individual goals are set for each member of the dyad in Session 1. In addition, on the TIQ-I, both partners need to comment on their own and each other's appraisal of their index trauma. Starting in Session 3, the therapist needs to identify situations avoided by each partner, some of which may be overlapping, to target in the *in vivo* approach assignments. The therapist should be careful to make sure that approach assignments are made for each partner as well as for the dyad. The communication skills and topics for the couple to discuss in Phase 2 remain unchanged in our delivery of the intervention given the mutual tone of the questions presented in the protocol. It should be noted that the dual-PTSD couple has generally done more cognitive assignments because of the increased number of potential stuck points that can be identified.

In delivering Phase 3 of the protocol, we have experimented with different ways of delivering the trauma-focused sessions. In early cases, we doubled the sessions, delivering two sessions per topic covered in Sessions 8–14 so that each partner had a dedicated session for his or her trauma-focused work. This seemed to work relatively well, but obviously lengthened the protocol by seven sessions for a total of 22. This length may or may not be acceptable to a given couple or to the particular setting in which the therapist works. With that prior success, we are currently testing the protocol in a series of case studies in which we deliver the 15-session protocol to dual-PTSD couples to determine whether we can successfully address both partners' trauma-related cognitions without doubling the number of treatment sessions in Phase 3. We are seeking to determine whether we can more efficiently deliver the intervention by first eliciting stuck points common to each partner and then targeting those stuck points that may not be common across partners. This approach is similar to that used in the group delivery of other trauma-focused interventions and the methods that we and others have used in delivering the protocol in multidyad groups.

## *Multidyad Groups*

There are a number of benefits to delivering the intervention in a multidyad group format, including the opportunity for vicarious learning, normalization of symptoms and relationship effects, increased social support beyond the dyad, and accountability to the group to do the in- and out-of-session practice. The intervention can be delivered in multiple ways. For example, several PTSD treatment teams and members of our training team have delivered CBCT for PTSD in groups comprising veterans and their intimate partners within U.S. VA medical centers. These teams have generally elected to deliver Phases 1 and 2 of the therapy in a multidyad group format. In collaboration with the National Center for Family Homelessness (*www.family-homelessness.org*), through funding provided by WalMart Corporation, we also have experience in delivering Phases 1 and 2 of the intervention in mixed groups of intimate and nonintimate dyads that included a service member or veteran.

Some clinicians have followed the delivery of Phases 1 and 2 in multidyad groups with the delivery of Phase 3 to individual dyads who are interested in doing the trauma-focused work in an individual couple therapy format. However, a few teams have opted to deliver the entire CBCT for PTSD protocol, including Phase 3 consisting of the trauma-focused cognitive processing, in the multidyad group context. Both of these approaches seem to have worked based on anecdotal report. We support both of these approaches to delivering Phase 3 based on available evidence and because the trauma-focused work is done from a cognitive perspective. Yet it is important to be aware that there is a greater likelihood of disclosure of details about traumatic events in the group if Phase 3 is delivered in addition to Phases 1 and 2. Similar to the delivery of any trauma-focused intervention in a group setting, clinicians should be especially vigilant about managing and processing trauma details shared in the multidyad group context.

To achieve maximum benefits from these groups, it is imperative that the group leaders (we recommend co-leaders for multidyad groups whenever possible) screen each dyad prior to inclusion in a group, using the inclusion/exclusion criteria reviewed earlier. It is our experience that the success of these groups is also dependent on the degree to which therapists collaboratively develop clear, definitive ground rules regarding confidentiality, not allow one member of the dyad to come without the other, require respectful communication and feedback to everyone within the group, and expect that the group will be notified by group members who will be absent. Like other skills-focused groups, the success of these groups hinges on good group process and closely adhering to the structure of the intervention.

Regardless of the number of therapy phases delivered in the group context, ground rules regarding the sharing of trauma details and the rationale for these rules should be clearly articulated. The expected reaction of the leaders to detailed trauma disclosure should be discussed (e.g., the leaders will immediately stop the speaker if the sharing becomes too detailed, gory, or gratuitous) to foster a sense of safety within the group.

When you deliver the intervention in groups, keep in mind that OOSA review must be done in a "sampling" manner: Not every aspect of the OOSAs completed by each dyad can be reviewed in each session. Rather, the group leaders must attempt to review OOSA completion equitably across dyads while making sure to shore up dyads who are struggling because of knowledge and/or motivation deficits. The leaders should look for themes in the responses or difficulties in completing the OOSAs to facilitate cohesion in the group and to maximize the power of the intervention across dyads. With regard to practice within session, leaders give the dyads time to practice the different communication skills together, and they rove among them to provide feedback and pick up on common difficulties found in their communication practice. The leaders can then troubleshoot and model for the group how to overcome these difficulties within the session. When doing the cognitive intervention, skilled leaders look for common stuck points to target to maximize the efficacy of the cognitive interventions in the group context.

## *Individual Delivery*

Our newest innovation is the delivery of therapy to individuals with traumatic stress who have intimate partners who are unable or unwilling to participate in the therapy sessions. In these cases, we have delivered the same interventions but with slight adaptation in their delivery. More specifically, we still deliver the psychoeducation from an interpersonal perspective, teach all of the communication skills, assign *in vivo* approach assignments, teach the interpersonally oriented cognitive strategy, and use this strategy for trauma-focused processing in Phase 3. We encourage patients receiving the therapy to teach their partner about what they are learning in the therapy and to invite their partner to participate in the interventions outside of session. However, we caution patients not to force or cajole their intimate partner into participation. Specific instructions in the OOSAs have been adapted for patients to invite their partner *once* to hear about what they have learned in session and to participate in the skills use outside of session. In a recent case, the intimate partner of a patient completed the TIQ-I after the patient provided him with information about what she had learned in Session 1. He completed the TIQ-I and provided excellent information on his perception of the effect of the trauma and related symptoms on their relationship and offered his own view on why his and his wife's son had died at birth. This provided the therapist with important information about the patient's relationship with her husband and about the husband's cognitions regarding their shared traumatic event.

Irrespective of partners' or others' interest or choice to use the skills, we encourage patients to practice the skills in these relationships with the rationale that their changes may effect change in the relational systems. Even if their changes do not cause improvements in the relationships, the patients can feel good that they are doing what they can to effect change. We encourage them to adopt a wait-and-see attitude about how interactions in these relationships might change based on their consistent use of the skills. The patients can also feel good about addressing their individual traumatic stress symptoms.

Within these treatment sessions, patients practice and model the various skills with the therapist. The *in vivo* approach assignments are still ideally constructed to double as shared rewarding activities with intimate partners if at all possible (e.g., going out to restaurants, movies, concerts). Patients are also educated to dissuade their loved ones from accommodating their avoidant behavior and to discuss alternative means for their partner to express love and concern if the accommodation also serves this function. With regard to the cognitive strategy, patients are encouraged to share the steps with their partner and/or trusted others for them to participate but are urged to use the process regardless of others' participation.

Just as in the conjoint application of the therapy, we conduct ongoing assessment of individual symptoms and relationship satisfaction across treatment. In the few cases where we have delivered the therapy in this individual format, mental health symptoms and relationship satisfaction have improved. Interestingly, it seems that the skills are being used across a wider range of relationships when delivered individually, perhaps because intimate partners are not in the room to define the skill use within that relationship context or because individuals who do not have an intimate partner willing/able to participate in the therapy rely more on other relationships. In any event, we look forward to accumulating more data on this format, with hopes that we might be able to expand the reach of the therapy to an even larger segment of individuals to improve individual and relational functioning after traumatic stress exposure.

## *Coordination with Other Interventions*

If a full course of CBCT for PTSD is not offered as a stand-alone intervention for traumatic stress problems, it is worth considering how loved ones can be involved in treatment in some way to improve the health and well-being of traumatized individuals. The phase-based nature of CBCT for PTSD lends itself well to meeting the goal of including loved ones in some manner in a treatment plan for traumatic stress problems. If the primary goal of including loved ones is to improve the effectiveness of individual treatment, psychoeducation for loved ones is a low-cost and usually powerful adjunct to existing individual therapies for traumatic stress problems. The interventions involved in Phase 1 (i.e., psychoeducation about symptoms and their maintenance/rationale for treatment, decreasing the most deleterious relationship behaviors and improving conflict resolution) might be used in conjunction with an evidence-based psychosocial or psychopharmacological treatment for PTSD to decrease the likelihood of treatment-interfering behavior on the part of loved ones and to decrease the most hostile and critical behaviors that have been found to negatively affect individually delivered treatment for PTSD.

With increasing willingness on the part of traumatized individuals and their loved ones to participate in treatment, and when there is relationship distress and/or accommodation of the symptoms on the part of concerned others (one or both are expected to be the prototypical presentation), Phase 2 of CBCT for PTSD could also be provided. This stage focuses on improving communication and problem-solving skills, decreasing behavioral and emotional avoidance, and introducing cognitive change facilitated by the inclusion of significant others. All of the interventions involved in Phase 2 of CBCT for PTSD are expected to be complementary to or to enhance current evidence-based psychotherapies for PTSD. For example, all of these therapies include a focus on decreasing avoidance and, to varying degrees, modifying appraisals that have caused or maintain the disorder. Phases 1 and 2 could also be used in conjunction with a plan that includes only medication or medication in conjunction with evidence-based psychotherapy. The interventions involved in Phases 1 and 2 can be easily delivered in a group setting, as discussed previously, or may be used when a traumatized individual and/or loved one does not wish to do trauma-focused work in the conjoint context or does not wish to commit to the full 15 sessions of CBCT for PTSD.

## Summary

We recommend that you consider the inclusion/exclusion criteria that have been used in prior trials of CBCT for PTSD in selecting couples who are an appropriate fit for CBCT for PTSD. These criteria are relatively inclusive but exclude individuals who are *acutely* psychotic, manic, suicidal, homicidal, ready to end their relationship, or severely aggressive and substance dependent (not abusing). In addition, objective assessment over the course of treatment allows clinicians to evaluate outcomes over time for the individual with PTSD and his or her loved one to better appreciate changes in symptoms and outcomes in their life and relationships.

Undoubtedly, you will work harder with couples who present with the types of clinical complications reviewed here, and you might even wonder whether the treatment can work for these kinds of cases. Based on our own experience and as discussed throughout this chapter, it is indeed possible to treat couples who present with one or more of these features and to observe improvements in both individual- and relationship-level outcomes. In fact, the structure of the therapy is often settling to the most distressed and disturbed patients and their partners and provides an alternative to the sense of hopelessness that can accompany years of trying to manage their difficulties without much success.

Given the severity and complexity of the presenting problem(s), the improvements might be more modest after a single round of therapy, but it does not mean that further improvement after the course of therapy is not possible: Couples just might need more time to practice the skills and consolidate gains. For couples who complete a full course of treatment as prescribed and still have clinically significant mental health or relationship problems, one option is to schedule a check-in or booster session 1 or 2 months after the last session. We have found this to be a powerful motivator for them to keep up with the skills learned during treatment and to reinforce the notion that they are well on their way to becoming their own helpers. In fact, in a number of cases treated in the context of our research studies, when we brought the couple back for a follow-up assessment several months later, the patient's PTSD and depressive symptoms had continued to decrease, the partner's own mental health continued to improve, and the couple's relationship adjustment continued to increase. For couples who have exerted reasonable efforts to continue working on issues but would like additional help addressing remaining problem areas following a break from therapy during which they keep working on their skills, it might be appropriate to consider contracting for further sessions using the skills on specific stuck points if there are residual issues after a full dose of the therapy. This approach is consistent with the notion of "episodes of care" and highlights your role as consultant, as the couple themselves are now the experts on their relationship.

Even if a full course of CBCT for PTSD is not used, phases of the therapy might be used to enhance individually delivered therapy for PTSD. Depending on the nature of the problems and a dyad's willingness to engage in trauma-focused therapy, different phases of the therapy can be used in the overall treatment plan for an individual with PTSD. Further research is needed to determine the relative benefit of this approach to treatment planning.

We find it extremely rewarding to see progress in the couples with whom we work and to watch them go through the healing process together. That said, it is especially gratifying to witness improvements in some of the most troubled patients and their partners and to have the privilege of joining them in the process of achieving these hard-won gains.

The next section contains the session-by session protocol comprising CBCT for PTSD.

# PART II

## CBCT FOR PTSD TREATMENT MANUAL

# PHASE 1

# Rationale for Treatment and Education about PTSD and Relationships

# SESSION 1

# Introduction to Treatment

---

**SUMMARY OF SESSION CONTENT**

*Goals*

- Provide an overview of the treatment course.
- Educate the couple about the symptoms of PTSD within an interpersonal context.
- Discuss the treatment rationale for CBCT for PTSD, introducing the concept of impeded recovery and the targets of the treatment to facilitate recovery.
- Develop goals with respect to improving both PTSD and the couple's relationship.
- Motivate the couple for completion of out-of-session assignments (OOSAs).

*Key Interventions*

1. Treatment Overview (*Cognitive-Behavioral Conjoint Therapy for PTSD: Session Overview, Handout 1.1*)
    - Time limited and in phases
    - Goals of treatment: improving relationships and decreasing PTSD symptoms
    - Out-of-session assignments
    - Increasing positivity
    - Conjoint therapy frame (limits of confidentiality)
2. Psychoeducation about PTSD: A Disorder of Impeded Recovery (*Cycle of PTSD Symptoms and Recovery from Trauma, Handout 1.2*)
    - Four clusters of PTSD symptoms
    - Dynamic association among symptoms and occurrence within intimate relationships
    - Natural versus impeded recovery
    - Therapy targets: cognitive and behavioral
3. Goal Setting/Treatment Contract (*Treatment Contract, Handout 1.3*)
    - Goals for both PTSD symptoms and intimate relationships
    - Goals that are behaviorally measurable
    - Goals that are realistic
4. Out-of-Session Assignments (*Handout 1.6*)
    - *Cycle of PTSD Symptoms and Recovery from Trauma* (Handout 1.2)
    - *Trauma and Relationships* (Handout 1.4)
    - *Trauma Impact Questions–I* (Handout 1.5—one copy for each partner)
    - *You've Been Caught Doing Something Nice* (Handout 1.6)
5. Check-Out

*Administer the patient and partner versions of PCL/relationship happiness.

## Treatment Overview

Distribute a copy of the *Cognitive-Behavioral Conjoint Therapy for PTSD: Session Overview* (*Handout 1.1*) for the couple to review as you provide an overview of the treatment.

### *Time-Limited Intervention and Therapy Phases*

The simultaneous goals of the therapy are to (1) improve the couple's relationship functioning and (2) decrease PTSD symptoms in one or both members. The therapy begins with a focus on making sure that both partners have a good working understanding of why we think people do not recover from traumatic events and, consequently, have PTSD and other comorbid conditions such as depression, general anxiety, and substance use disorders. The psychoeducation also addresses the ways in which the couple's interactions and structure can contribute to the nonrecovery of the traumatized person and why we believe the couple's relationship holds such promise in ameliorating PTSD symptoms. The first phase of therapy includes a focus on immediately increasing positive affect and behavior in the couple through specific behavioral exercises and better managing conflict in the relationship in order to decrease the deleterious effects of these behaviors.

The second phase of therapy focuses on improving the couple's relationship functioning through enhanced communication both to increase satisfaction and to facilitate trauma-focused dyadic cognitive interventions in Phase 3. This phase of therapy also has the goal of modifying couple behaviors that maintain and contribute to emotional and behavioral avoidance on the part of the person with PTSD and potentially his or her partner.

The final phase is designed to capitalize on the improvements from the first two phases of the therapy to address specific cognitions about the traumatic event and its consequences that have prevented the traumatized person from recovering from trauma(s) and that may be maintaining relationship distress. Consistent with the conjoint therapy frame adopted in this therapy, cognitions held by both partners are targeted and collaboratively explored. These cognitions have overlapping interpersonal and intimate relationship functioning implications (e.g., trust, emotional intimacy). Partners' cognitions that may contribute to difficulties in recovery are also targeted (e.g., "She is too fragile to handle talking about difficult topics").

The following is an example of the explanation of the therapy structure and phases:

*Today is our first session of the therapy, and I would like to spend most of this time getting to know you and explaining the goals of the therapy we will be doing together. We'll discuss some of the techniques that you will be learning when we work together. I'll be doing more of the talking in this session compared with future sessions.*

*The therapy consists of 15 sessions, each lasting 75 minutes. In this therapy, there are two parallel treatment goals: (1) to improve your relationship and (2) to decrease PTSD symptoms in one or both of you.*

*There are three phases of the therapy we will be doing together.*

1. ***Phase 1. Rationale for Treatment and Education.*** *The initial portion of therapy will involve discussion about the symptoms of PTSD, why we think people do not recover from traumatic events, and how trauma has impacted each of you and your relationship. We will also talk about the healing power of your relationship in helping _____ recover and make meaning of his/her trauma(s). In this phase of therapy, we will also explore how **avoidance** of all kinds of different emotions, situations, relationships, memories, and thoughts poorly impacts relationships. It is quite common for people to want to escape or avoid memories, situations, thoughts, and feelings that are painful and distressing to them. However, while the strategy of avoiding painful experiences works in the short run, it actually maintains or worsens PTSD and relationship problems in the long run.*

2. ***Phase 2. Satisfaction Enhancement and Undermining Avoidance.*** *The next phase in building a solid foundation will be to **increase the satisfaction** in your relationship and improve the ways that you deal with conflict in your relationship. Communication problems are **the** most often cited problems for couples. We will work on specific skills that you can use to improve the way you talk with each other. We focus on these skills early because without these skills it is difficult to communicate successfully about specific core beliefs that are keeping your PTSD and relationship problems in place. In this phase of therapy, we will also actively search for ways in which your relationship contributes to avoidance or ways in which your relationship can help **undermine avoidance** that maintains your PTSD and relationship problems.*

3. ***Phase 3. Making Meaning of the Trauma(s) and Ending the Therapy.*** *In the last phase of our work together, we will use your enhanced relationship skills to explore and reconsider the ways that each of you have made meaning of the traumatic event and your relationship in order to continue to improve PTSD and your relationship. Making healthier, more accurate meaning of traumatic events and your relationship will help you feel less anxious, depressed, angry, guilty, and/or ashamed as individuals and to feel closer and happier in your relationship. We will be working on **both** of your thoughts and beliefs that contribute to relationship problems and PTSD symptoms. This phase of therapy includes the **end of therapy** but a commitment to ongoing work on yourselves and your relationship.*

## *Out-of-Session Assignments and Increasing Positivity*

*After each session, you will have an out-of-session assignment to help you practice the skills you have learned in our sessions. This is designed to get the therapy out of this therapy room and into your life. Like everything, the more that you practice these skills in your everyday life, the more you will gain from the therapy.*

*One of the first assignments will be to increase the positive interactions between the two of you. We know that to improve relationships it is not enough to just get rid of the bad; we must also add in good. Throughout the therapy, I am going to ask that you put your best foot forward—pull out all the stops to try and improve yourself and your relationship—so that you can know that you did the best you could.*

*Does that make sense to you?*

## Conjoint Therapy Frame

As discussed in Part I, CBCT for PTSD is inherently systemic in its conceptualization of individual and couple functioning. We conceptualize individuals with PTSD to exist in a dynamic and interactional couple system that reinforces or diminishes individual psychopathology. Each member of the couple is conceptualized to co-create their relationship successes and problems and mutually influence their individual functioning.

For both theoretical and pragmatic reasons, it is important that the couple at least understands and, it is hoped, endorses the conjoint model. Theoretically, the conjoint frame is important to avoiding the potential that one member of the couple is identified as the "problem partner" or "identified patient." In this setting, the couple, and more specifically their communication and interacting belief systems, is the patient. Pragmatically, adhering to the conjoint therapy frame is important to avoiding any potential triangulation or compromising confidentiality issues as well as decreasing the risk of pathologizing the traumatized individual.

> *In this couple therapy, we consider the "patient" to be your relationship. More specifically, your ways of communicating with each other, and the ways that your individual thoughts and beliefs interact with one another, are the focus of this therapy. Although one or both of you is diagnosed with PTSD, neither of you is the patient identified to be fixed. Rather, we consider your individual problems to exist in a relationship that has the potential to improve each of you as individuals. In other words, each of you impacts the other in your interactions, and those interactions have the potential for individual improvements. Both of you will be responsible for improving your relationship, which will improve each of you.*
>
> *A natural consequence of our couple focus is that all of the information that we discuss will be kept within our couple sessions. There are a few situations in which I am required by law to break confidentiality (e.g., child abuse/neglect, elder abuse/neglect, subpoena, imminent danger to self or other). Otherwise, what we talk about here is confidential.*
>
> *Our work will be intensive and you may find that you are experiencing discomfort as we discuss certain topics, feelings, situations, and so on. I want you to know that I would be happy to talk with you as a couple between sessions if you feel that you cannot cope with your feelings alone. However, without both of you present, I will avoid talking about issues related to your therapy. This is to avoid any miscommunications and to make sure no one feels as though he or she has been left out of important discussions and decisions.*
>
> *What concerns do you have about this couple focus?*

## Psychoeducation about PTSD: A Disorder of Impeded Recovery

It is important for both members of the couple to have an understanding of the nature of PTSD, its symptom clusters, and how these clusters are dynamically connected to each other. It is helpful to begin with the *reexperiencing* cluster of symptoms and discuss how the reexperiencing of traumatic events leads to *hyperarousal* symptoms. When faced with traumatic reminders of events and the hyperarousal and distress related to reminders, people often want to *avoid* those reminders (e.g., memories, people, places, things). People may also avoid their feelings by *emotionally numbing* them. In our experience, it is extremely important that the couple leave the session understanding the negative feedback loop that exists because of avoidance and emotion numbing. **With behavioral avoidance and emotional numbing, clients and their loved ones are deprived of new learning. For example, they do not learn that a plastic sack on the side of the road is just a plastic sack and not an improvised explosive device. They do not learn that the scent of a certain cologne does not foretell sexual assault.** This is imperative for the couple's buy-in to complete *in vivo* approach activities, increase emotional experiencing and expression in their relationship, and engage in trauma-focused cognitive work. It is crucial to the rationale for conducting this trauma-focused therapy. The *Cycle of PTSD Symptoms and Recovery from Trauma (Handout 1.2)* is used to reinforce this point.

Compared with psychoeducation about PTSD that might be delivered in an individual therapy format, there are two important differences in CBCT for PTSD. First, it is important to discuss behavioral avoidance symptoms separate from emotional numbing symptoms. Taxometric research supports this differentiation (e.g., Asmundson et al., 2004; King, Leskin, King, & Weathers, 1998), and because emotional numbing is particularly detrimental for couple functioning, we identify these two different types of symptoms. Second, the symptoms of PTSD should be presented within an interpersonal context. In other words, how do these symptoms manifest in the couple's relationship? How do these symptoms affect the couple? Walk the couple through the symptom clusters illustrated on the handout. We recommend that you begin the psychoeducation by asking the couple what they know about the symptoms of PTSD and its treatment to get a sense of their level of knowledge and also to correct any misconceptions about the disorder (e.g., that it is not possible to recover from PTSD).

*It is important that, as a couple, you have a good understanding of PTSD. PTSD encompasses four different types of symptoms: reexperiencing, behavioral avoidance, emotional numbing, and hyperarousal symptoms.*

- *__Reexperiencing:__ The common factor in reexperiencing symptoms is that the person with PTSD routinely "reexperiences" the traumatic event(s) in some way. This can be through unwanted thoughts or images, nightmares, flashbacks, and psychological distress or physiological distress when reminded of traumatic events.*

  *What reexperiencing symptoms have you noticed? How have they affected your relationship (e.g., sleeping in separate beds because of nightmares, partner intervention during a flashback; partner interrupting traumatic memory with grounding)?*

- *__Hyperarousal:__ As a result of chronically reexperiencing the traumatic event(s), the body is in a chronic state of hyperarousal. It is very adaptive for survival to have the fight-or-flight response whenever there is danger. This very automatic response prepares the body to fight or flee when in danger. However, chronically being in a state of fighting or fleeing is very taxing on the mind and body. This hyperarousal state is seen in sleep disturbance, irritability/anger, concentration problems, hypervigilance, and exaggerated startle.*

*Which hyperarousal symptoms have you each noticed? How have they affected your relationship (e.g., verbal or physical aggression, hostility, difficulty communicating because of concentration problems, sleeping in separate beds because of sleep disturbance, controlling behaviors because of hypervigilance)?*

• ***Avoidance:*** *Individuals with PTSD seek to avoid reminders of traumatic events in order to avoid the unpleasant feelings associated with them (e.g., anxiety, guilt, shame, anger). These triggers may be people, places, or things. There also tends to be avoidance of thoughts and feelings. Individuals with PTSD can avoid through many means, such as alcohol/drugs, sex, workaholism, gambling, or self-injury.*

*What signs of avoidance you have noticed? How has avoidance played out in your relationship (e.g., sex, substance use, not going out to busy places, avoiding family gatherings)?*

• ***Emotional Numbing:*** *People who have been exposed to a traumatic event may feel extremely afraid, helpless, or horrified. Sometimes these feelings are overwhelming, and, in order to cope they may disconnect from them for a temporary decrease in their intensity. In cases when people are faced with a very dangerous or intensely frightening situation, emotional numbing can serve as a very adaptive response. The "freezing" response is adaptive when a situation is inescapable and out of the person's control. The body protectively becomes still and "hunkers down" for anticipated injury. Over time, emotional numbing can become a learned response to cope with a variety of stressful or uncomfortable situations because people feel less anxious or distressed in the moment. However, as a result of this way of coping with stress in the long term, individuals with PTSD do not get to learn that they are actually safe in the here and now and can tolerate their own anxiety or discomfort. An unintended consequence of emotional numbing is that, while it numbs people to negative feelings, it also desensitizes them to feel positive emotions.*

*Tell me about signs of emotional numbing. In what ways has this affected your relationship (e.g., difficulties with communication, feeling emotionally and/or physically disconnected)?*

*These symptoms feed on one another, creating a loop that maintains and can even worsen symptoms. Avoidance or numbing prevents new learning. You are deprived of new information from your experiences—you don't learn that things that remind you of the trauma may not be actual signs of danger. A primary goal of our work together is to stop that loop.*

Compared with other mental health disorders, PTSD does not *develop* per se. Rather, in the immediate aftermath of a traumatic event, most people will have symptoms of PTSD. In the majority those symptoms subside with time, giving way to a *natural recovery*. For some, however, the PTSD symptoms do not subside, and they are diagnosed with PTSD (Riggs et al., 1995; Rothbaum et al., 1992). It is most appropriate to think of PTSD as a disorder of impeded recovery from a traumatic event and to conceptualize the patient as having barriers or impediments to recovery. What got in the way of this patient recovering from the traumatic event? Convey to the couple this understanding of PTSD and refer to *Cycle of PTSD Symptoms and Recovery from Trauma* (Handout 1.2).

Explain to the couple that there are a variety of reasons why some people do not recover from a traumatic event. In CBCT for PTSD, we use two classes of interventions to facilitate recovery:

1. ***Behavioral interventions*** to address *avoidance* of trauma-related reminders and internal experiences (e.g., memories, thoughts, feelings) and *emotional numbing*.
2. ***Cognitive interventions*** to address *problematic appraisals of traumatic event(s)* (e.g., unrealistic self- or other-blame, hindsight bias) and *maladaptive here-and-now beliefs* about the self, others, and the world that emanate from trauma(s).

*There are a number of reasons why some people do not experience a natural recovery after a traumatic event. In this therapy, we use two types of interventions to target the biggest and changeable impediments to recovery. One is avoidance. As long as you avoid, you never get a chance to learn that you are safe in the here and now, and you reinforce the belief that you are still in danger. Avoidance also prevents you from looking back on the trauma with enough detail so that you can make sense of why it happened. A second impediment is emotional numbing. Although it looks different from behavioral avoidance, emotional numbing functions in a similar way: to decrease uncomfortable feelings. As long as you numb out, it reinforces the belief that you can't tolerate feeling whatever emotion you're having. To help address avoidance and emotional numbing, we will work on helping the two of you to communicate better and to approach, rather than avoid, the things that make you feel uncomfortable about.*

*The third impediment is the way you think about the event. Both of you have drawn certain conclusions about how the world works, and some of those conclusions can get in the way of you moving forward with your life and relating to each other in the ways that you would like to. For instance, you may believe that the traumas that you (or your loved one) have experienced are your fault and that you have to keep your guard up and control everything in an attempt to prevent bad things from happening to you and those you care about. Alternatively, you may blame others and now believe that you can't trust anyone ever again. Because of the avoidance, you've never had a chance to consider other ways of seeing the event, and because of the emotional numbing, you've never had a chance to learn that you can handle uncomfortable feelings.*

*In our work together, we're going to use your relationship to decrease this avoidance and emotional numbing and to consider new ways of seeing the event, yourself, and other people. In essence, we are going to use your relationship to remove these barriers so that your own process of natural recovery can kick in.*

## Goal Setting/Treatment Contract

Keeping in mind the parallel and overarching goals of this therapy to decrease PTSD symptoms and improve relationship functioning, develop specific goals for treatment in collaboration with the couple. At least one goal should focus on PTSD-related symptomatology (e.g., better anger management, less guilt, less reexperiencing, less numbing), and one goal should focus on relationship functioning (e.g., specific areas of better communication and intimacy, less fighting). These goals are likely to be interconnected.

Encourage the couple to be as specific as possible when setting their goals. This is especially important when urging them to articulate what they might notice if there are improvements (i.e., specific behaviors observed, based on goals identified in the *Treatment Contract, Handout 1.3*). For example, ask the couple, "How will you know that you are more intimate with each other?" Specific behaviors might include holding hands more often, saying "I love you" more often, hugging more frequently, increased sexual experiences, or increased sharing of feelings.

*Figure 1.1* provides an example of relationship- and PTSD-oriented goals for a sexual assault survivor and her partner. Susan and Jake, the couple from Chapter 2, identified a number of goals in each domain and, with the therapist's coaching, were able to make abstract goals behaviorally specific. For instance, in the relationship domain, they identified the goal of less hostility, which would be evident in the form of no name calling and decreased sarcasm toward each other. They also listed the goal of increased intimacy, which would be noticeable in the form of more hand holding and sexual contact. With regard to improvements in PTSD symptoms, they specified the goal of decreased flashbacks, which would be apparent in the form of Susan's being able to hear punk rock music and not feeling as if she were reliving the rape. They also named the goal of decreased avoidance. When the therapist asked how they would know

| Our goals: | What we will observe (behavioral): |
|---|---|
| **1. Improve our relationship** | |
| *Better communication* | *Less arguing* |
| *Less hostility* | *No name calling; less sarcasm toward each other* |
| *Increased intimacy* | *More hand holding and sexual contact* |
| *More fun together* | *More date (e.g., movies) and hiking* |
| **2. Improve PTSD symptoms** | |
| *Decreased flashbacks* | *Hear punk rock music and not feel as if back there* |
| *Decreased hypervigilance* | *No checking locks on doors and windows* |
| *Decreased avoidance* | *Go to bars, concerts; physical touch of all kinds* |
| *Decreased numbing* | *Feel love, joy, anger, sadness, fear* |
| | |
| | |
| | |

**FIGURE 1.1.** Susan and Jake's relationship- and PTSD-oriented goals.

Susan was avoiding less, they stated that they as a couple would go to bars and concerts, which they had heretofore avoided, and engage in physical touch of all kinds.

Make sure that the couple's goals are realistic. In this vein, it is important to steer the couple toward developing goals that mark **improvement, not perfection**. It is important to convey to the couple that relationship perfection is impossible to attain. Like all couples, they will still have relationship problems and issues that arise even after completing the treatment. The idea is that they will be able to resolve those problems more efficiently and effectively. Similarly, you should highlight the notion that individual stress and problems wax and wane over time. The goal is to find *improvements* in both PTSD and relationship functioning and a greater capacity to deal with problems as they arise in the future.

If there is low-level aggression occurring in the relationship, both partners should agree that these are unhelpful methods of resolving conflict or managing anger. They should be explicitly asked to make a commitment to each other and the therapist to stop these behaviors. Point out that the interventions they will be receiving in the course of the therapy will help them honor this commitment. A simple written contract can be used to aid in keeping their commitment. If commitments cannot be made or you question the couple's ability to comply with their commitments, the therapy may be delayed until a time at which the couple can successfully make these commitments.

Record the couple's goals on the *Treatment Contract* (*Handout 1.3*). Have each partner witness the signature of the other.

## Out-of-Session Assignments

Orient the couple to the OOSA summary (*Handout 1.6*) for this session and point out the following assignments:

- Ask the couple to review the *Cycle of PTSD Symptoms and Recovery from Trauma* (*Handout 1.2*) **together** prior to the next session.
- Ask the couple to read *Trauma and Relationships* (*Handout 1.4*) **together** prior to the next session.
- Request that **each partner** complete the *Trauma Impact Questions–I* (*Handout 1.5*). Inform the couple that this will be important information to use in the next session as they understand PTSD and its connection to relationship functioning. *Their responses will be read aloud at the next session.* They can share them with each other beforehand if they want to. It is important to stress that this is not a trauma account. Rather, the assignment is designed to help the couple and the therapist better understand how they each made meaning of events and how they construe themselves and their relationship.
- Remind the couple that to increase relationship satisfaction they must not only decrease the negative aspects of their relationship but also *increase* the positive aspects. The OOSA You've Been Caught Doing Something Nice (*Handout 1.6*) is designed to address this. Each partner is asked to notice, on a daily basis, when the other does something nice for him or her. This can be a big or a small act, but the smaller the better. Each partner should comment on this noticed behavior to the other and record the specific behavior on the form *each day*. Preemptively, note that the couple might be tempted to

complete the assignment only the night before or the day of the next session. Point out the advantages of positive exchanges more consistently over the time between sessions. Also encourage the couple to put the form in a place where they both can see it.

## Check-Out

Reserve several minutes at the end of the session to ask each member of the couple how the session worked for them. Also, inquire of each what they would like to take with them from the session.

HANDOUT 1.1

# Cognitive-Behavioral Conjoint Therapy for PTSD
*Session Overview*

**R.E.S.U.M.E. LIVING**

**Phase 1. Rationale for Treatment and Education about PTSD and Relationships**

    Session 1.   Introduction to Treatment

    Session 2.   Safety Building

**Phase 2. Satisfaction Enhancement and Undermining Avoidance**

    Session 3.   Listening and Approaching

    Session 4.   Sharing Thoughts and Feelings: Emphasis on *Feelings*

    Session 5.   Sharing Thoughts and Feelings: Emphasis on *Thoughts*

    Session 6.   Getting U.N.S.T.U.C.K.

    Session 7.   Problem Solving to Shrink PTSD

**Phase 3. Making Meaning of the Trauma(s) and End of Therapy**

    Session 8.   Acceptance

    Session 9.   Blame

    Session 10. Trust

    Session 11. Control

    Session 12. Emotional Closeness

    Session 13. Physical Closeness

    Session 14. Posttraumatic Growth

    Session 15. Review and Reinforcement of Treatment Gains

---

From *Cognitive-Behavioral Conjoint Therapy for PTSD: Harnessing the Healing Power of Relationships* by Candice M. Monson and Steffany J. Fredman. Copyright 2012 by The Guilford Press. Permission to photocopy this handout is granted to purchasers of this book for personal use only (see copyright page for details).

HANDOUT 1.2

# Cycle of PTSD Symptoms and Recovery from Trauma

## Cycle of PTSD Symptoms

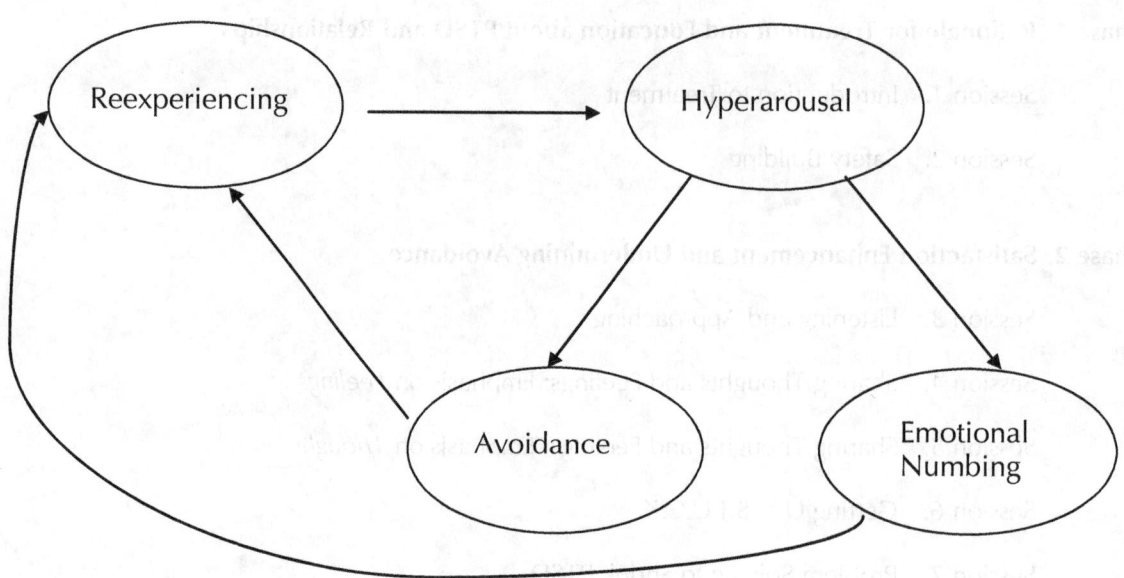

## Natural Recovery versus PTSD

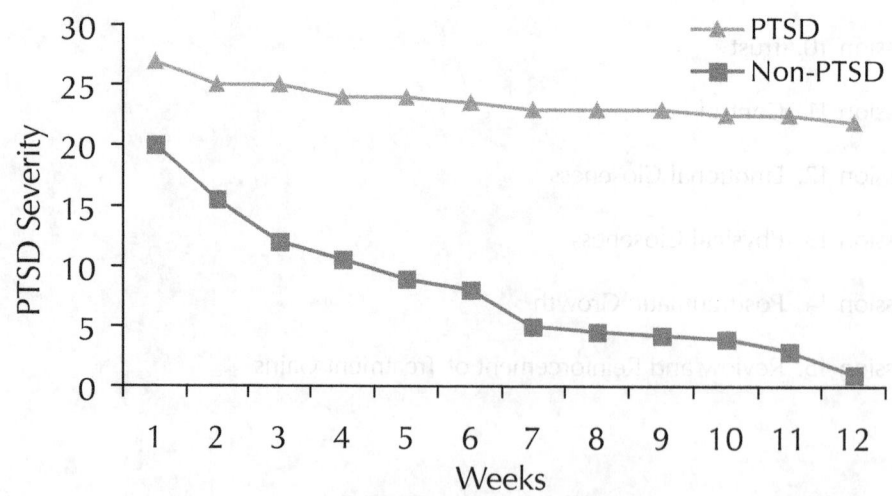

---

From *Cognitive-Behavioral Conjoint Therapy for PTSD: Harnessing the Healing Power of Relationships* by Candice M. Monson and Steffany J. Fredman. Copyright 2012 by The Guilford Press. Permission to photocopy this handout is granted to purchasers of this book for personal use only (see copyright page for details).

## HANDOUT 1.3

# Treatment Contract

### TREATMENT COMPONENTS—THREE PHASES

R = *Rationale* for Treatment  } Phase 1
E = *Education* about PTSD and Relationships

S = *Satisfaction* Enhancement  } Phase 2
U = *Undermining* Avoidance

M = *Making Meaning* of the Trauma(s)  } Phase 3
E = *End* of Therapy—commitment to ongoing betterment

Living

### TREATMENT EXPECTATIONS

1. Come to sessions as a couple
2. Keep information within conjoint sessions
3. Time limited
4. Out-of-session assignments to apply skills
5. Best foot forward
6. Focus on improving *both* your relationship *and* PTSD
7. Treatment targets: behavior and cognition

*(cont.)*

---

From *Cognitive-Behavioral Conjoint Therapy for PTSD: Harnessing the Healing Power of Relationships* by Candice M. Monson and Steffany J. Fredman. Copyright 2012 by The Guilford Press. Permission to photocopy this handout is granted to purchasers of this book for personal use only (see copyright page for details).

# Treatment Contract *(page 2 of 2)*

Our goals:                                What we will observe (behavioral):

**1. Improve our relationship**

_____            _____
_____            _____
_____            _____
_____            _____
_____            _____
_____            _____
_____            _____

**2. Improve PTSD symptoms**

_____            _____
_____            _____
_____            _____
_____            _____
_____            _____
_____            _____
_____            _____

I have read and received information regarding the therapy we are undertaking together and commit optimistically to myself and my partner to this and our goals listed above.

_____            _____
Partner                                   Date

_____            _____
Partner                                   Date

HANDOUT 1.4

# Trauma and Relationships

Exposure to a traumatic experience can cause both individual and relationship problems. Not all trauma reactions are the same, and you or your loved ones' reactions may be different from those of other people. This handout discusses some of the widespread reactions survivors and their loved ones can have after a traumatic event. You've been asked to read it together as a couple. As you review it, assess your feelings, thoughts, and actions and how they may be different since the traumatic experience.

## PTSD AS IMPEDED RECOVERY

A traumatic event exposes a person to a situation that is life-threatening or involves risk of bodily injury to him- or herself or someone else. Intense feelings are natural reactions to being faced with this kind of threat. For many people, these feelings and reactions related to the trauma decrease over the weeks and months after the trauma is over. Feeling those natural feelings, getting support from others, facing the memories and reminders of the trauma, and developing healthy thoughts about why the trauma occurred help people recover naturally from their trauma. However, in the case of posttraumatic stress disorder (PTSD), these feelings may persist because the person continues to think he or she is in danger, despite actually being physically safe.

There are two major reasons people experience PTSD, and we specifically target these two reasons in the therapy.

1. *Thinking about the trauma.* One reason people continue to have intense feelings and other difficulties in the wake of trauma is that they find it hard to make sense of the event and how or why it happened. This causes the trauma survivor to relive or reexperience the event in an attempt to understand and make sense of it. It is as if the person's mind is trying to fit the pieces of a puzzle together but hasn't quite figured out how to do this. As a result of constantly reliving the event, it makes the person feel as if the trauma is still happening. When reminded of the event, the person feels the same feelings he or she felt at the time of the event, and this causes him or her to feel unsafe in the present. Many things can trigger or prompt these memories and reactions to them—certain places, times of day, smells, sounds, people, emotions, and bodily sensations. Partners or other family members can also serve as triggers, particularly if the traumatic event was at the hands of another person (e.g., rape, robbery, combat).

2. *Avoiding and numbing.* The second reason people have PTSD is that they avoid those reminders and their feelings, which makes them feel better in the short run but has the negative consequences in the long run of maintaining the cycle of symptoms. In the long run, they do not get the opportunity to learn that these reminders and feelings do not necessarily signal danger.

## SYMPTOMS OF PTSD AND RELATIONSHIPS

PTSD consists of four different clusters of symptoms that feed off of one another to keep you stuck with the symptoms and relationship difficulties.

*(cont.)*

From *Cognitive-Behavioral Conjoint Therapy for PTSD: Harnessing the Healing Power of Relationships* by Candice M. Monson and Steffany J. Fredman. Copyright 2012 by The Guilford Press. Permission to photocopy this handout is granted to purchasers of this book for personal use only (see copyright page for details).

# Trauma and Relationships *(page 2 of 3)*

## *Reexperiencing Symptoms*

The reexperiencing symptoms of PTSD can take the form of unwanted or intrusive thoughts about the trauma, some of which can interfere with attention and concentration. In addition to fear, these memories can be associated with other negative emotions, such as anger, sadness, shame, and intense physiological reactions, such as racing heart, sweating, nausea, or stomach upset. Partners sometimes think the traumatized individual is not interested in or paying attention to what he or she is saying when, in fact, the person may be distracted by trauma memories and the distress associated with them. Trauma survivors can also have flashbacks or vivid images, leaving them feeling as if they are back in the event. Partners may try to cover up or explain away this reaction if the flashback occurs when other people are around. Bad dreams about the trauma are also common, and couples may find it hard to sleep in the same bed due to the traumatized individual's disturbed sleep and restlessness.

## *Hyperarousal Symptoms*

As a result of feeling like he or she is constantly reliving the event, the trauma survivor's fight-or-flight response is chronically activated. We are evolutionarily wired to fight or flee our way out of a situation that is truly dangerous in the moment, and then when we are no longer in danger, for the fight-or-flight response to turn off, like a light switch. However, in the case of PTSD, it is as though the light switch is on all the time with the trauma survivor feeling as if the trauma is still happening or that something bad is going to happen again. Being chronically in the fight-or-flight mode results in the hyperarousal (i.e., overaroused) symptoms of PTSD. These symptoms include anger and irritability, which can erode happiness in intimate relationships. Partners may sometimes feel they are "walking on eggshells" to avoid the traumatized individual becoming angry or agitated. As a result, couples and family members may find it hard to communicate, particularly when there are differences of opinions or preferences. Verbal and physical aggression have also been associated with these symptoms.

Other symptoms of hyperarousal include trouble sleeping, concentration problems, being easily startled, and being super-alert or hypervigilant. Traumatized individuals are hypervigilant to protect themselves and their loved ones from perceived danger, and this can take many forms. For instance, to be able to scan the environment for threat and keep himself and others safe, the trauma survivor may try to sit with his back to the wall rather than the door, frequently check door locks, sleep with the lights on, patrol the perimeter of the house for intruders, or call loved ones multiple times in a row to make sure that nothing bad has happened to them. This hypervigilance for threat can also extend to loved ones to the extent that the trauma survivor perceives the partner as critical or negative even though the partner does not feel this way. For example, leaving socks on the floor can be interpreted as a sign of disrespect or asking a question about why the trauma survivor was late for dinner could be interpreted as an accusation of infidelity.

## *Behavioral Avoidance*

Because it is unpleasant to reexperience a traumatic event and the hyperarousal that goes with the distressing memories, it is understandable that traumatized individuals might use a variety of strategies to feel better in the moment. One strategy is avoidance. Individuals with PTSD seek to avoid reminders of the traumatic event in their environment (such as people, places or things) and to avoid the unpleasant feelings associated with the event (e.g., anxiety, sadness, anger, guilt, shame). There also tends to be avoidance of thoughts and feelings associated with the reminders as well. Individuals with PTSD can avoid in many ways, including alcohol and drugs, sex, overworking, gambling, self-harm behaviors, and suicidal thinking. In an effort to be supportive, loved ones may try to protect or buffer traumatized

*(cont.)*

# Trauma and Relationships *(page 3 of 3)*

individuals from situations that make them feel anxious or otherwise uncomfortable, and couples may adapt their relationship to minimize the traumatized individual's discomfort. For example, as a couple, they may not do activities that involve being around groups of people or in open spaces because the traumatized individual feels exposed and vulnerable.

## *Emotional Numbing*

Emotional numbing is another way people who have been traumatized decrease the distress associated with trauma reminders. When people have been exposed to a traumatic event and feel extremely afraid, helpless, or horrified, they can feel overwhelmed and, to cope, disconnect from their feelings to temporarily decrease their intensity. Numbing is related to the freeze response, which occurs when the individual is in a life-threatening or otherwise intensely frightening situation and cannot fight or flee his or her way out of it. As a way of surviving, the body protectively becomes still and "hunkers down" for anticipated injury. In the case of PTSD, disconnecting from one's feelings becomes a general strategy to cope with a variety of stressful or uncomfortable situations so the individual can feel less anxious or distressed in the moment. In many cases, the emotional numbing happens almost automatically, and the traumatized individual may not even be aware that he or she is doing it.

Emotional numbing symptoms include difficulty feeling a range of emotions, both negative (e.g., anxiety, sadness, anger) and positive (e.g., joy, love). It is also seen through loss of interest in activities and people and feeling distant or cut off from others. Emotional numbing is particularly hard on intimate relationships because emotions serve as the "glue" that bonds people together. Emotions help couples feel close and connected to one another, and when they are not shared, partners can feel distant and disconnected.

Avoidance and numbing can contribute to problems with sexual relationships after a trauma. Sex, physical intimacy, and feeling vulnerable with another person more generally may be a trauma reminder and increase the urge to avoid or feel numb. Emotional numbing can contribute to difficulties feeling sexually interested due to lack of desire and difficulty feeling positive feelings, regardless of whether the trauma was sexual in nature. Physical closeness (sexual intimacy and physical affection more generally) is one way partners feel close to one another. When physical contact is uncomfortable or distressing for at least one person, couples may feel distant or cut off from one another.

## OTHER TRAUMA-RELATED PROBLEMS AND RELATIONSHIPS

Other problems that can occur after a trauma include guilt, shame, and depression. Trauma survivors sometimes feel guilty about or ashamed of things that they did or did not do at the time of the event and think negative thoughts about themselves, including thoughts that they can't trust themselves. They may also have trouble trusting other people, which can get in the way of feeling close to others. Negative thoughts about oneself and others can contribute to depression. When people are depressed, they feel sad and may lose interest in things that they used to enjoy or think were important, including work, hobbies, or spending time with loved ones. Sometimes, the depression can contribute to people thinking life isn't worth living and that they would be better off dead. These kinds of thoughts may function like avoidance in that they provide a way for the person to minimize his or her distress in the moment by thinking of death as an escape from the current pain and suffering. At times, a couple's relationship may be affected as well because the traumatized individual has withdrawn and the couple is not engaged in doing things as a couple.

HANDOUT 1.5

# Trauma Impact Questions–I

Name: _____

1. How has trauma or PTSD affected our relationship to date? How has it impacted my thoughts, feelings, and behaviors about our relationship?

_____
_____
_____
_____
_____
_____
_____
_____
_____
_____

2. Why did the traumatic event(s) happen to me or my partner?

_____
_____
_____
_____
_____
_____
_____
_____
_____
_____

*(cont.)*

---

From *Cognitive-Behavioral Conjoint Therapy for PTSD: Harnessing the Healing Power of Relationships* by Candice M. Monson and Steffany J. Fredman. Copyright 2012 by The Guilford Press. Permission to photocopy this handout is granted to purchasers of this book for personal use only (see copyright page for details).

## Trauma Impact Questions–I *(page 2 of 2)*

3. What do I believe in each of the following areas, as it relates to *me, my partner, and others*?

   **Trust:**

   _____
   _____
   _____
   _____

   **Control:**

   _____
   _____
   _____
   _____

   **Emotional Closeness:**

   _____
   _____
   _____
   _____

   **Physical Closeness:**

   _____
   _____
   _____
   _____

HANDOUT 1.6

# Out-of-Session Assignments
## Session 1. Introduction to Treatment

1. Review the *Cycle of PTSD Symptoms and Recovery from Trauma* (Handout 1.2) together prior to the next session.

2. Read the *Trauma and Relationships* (Handout 1.4) together at least once prior to the next session.

3. Each of you should complete the *Trauma Impact Questions–I* (Handout 1.5).

4. Each day, catch your partner doing something nice, and let him or her know that you have noticed this positive attitude and/or behavior. Place this form in an obvious place for the two of you and record on the form what you have noticed **each day**. Bring this form with you to the next session.

**Next appointment:** _____ @ _____.

## YOU'VE BEEN CAUGHT DOING SOMETHING NICE

Week of: _____

|           | Person Caught: | Person Caught: |
|-----------|----------------|----------------|
| Sunday    |                |                |
| Monday    |                |                |
| Tuesday   |                |                |
| Wednesday |                |                |
| Thursday  |                |                |
| Friday    |                |                |
| Saturday  |                |                |

---

From *Cognitive-Behavioral Conjoint Therapy for PTSD: Harnessing the Healing Power of Relationships* by Candice M. Monson and Steffany J. Fredman. Copyright 2012 by The Guilford Press. Permission to photocopy this handout is granted to purchasers of this book for personal use only (see copyright page for details).

# SESSION 2

# Safety Building

---

**SUMMARY OF SESSION CONTENT**

### Goals

- Increase emotional and physical (in some cases) safety in the relationship.
- Discuss disclosure of traumatic material in the relationship context.
- Decrease negative, hostile, and critical behavior in the relationship as quickly as possible, because negative behaviors have relatively greater impact on satisfaction than do positive behaviors.
- Increase relationship satisfaction and increase the likelihood that the couple can approach difficult topics surrounding traumatic experiences and their relationship in a manner that facilitates recovery by making relationship environment feel physically and emotionally safer.

### Key Interventions

1. Review of Out-of-Session Assignments
    - *Cycle of PTSD Symptoms and Recovery from Trauma (Handout 1.2)*
    - *You've Been Caught Doing Something Nice (Handout 1.6)*
    - *Trauma and Relationships (Handout 1.4)*
    - *Trauma Impact Questions–I (Handout 1.5)*
2. Trauma Focus and Disclosure
    - Explain the purpose of the index traumatic event.
    - Discussion around disclosure of specific traumatic information.
    - Address the couple's concerns.
3. Addressing Negative Behaviors as Barriers to Safety
    - Psychoeducation regarding negative relationship behaviors and PTSD.
    - Address safety issues within the relationship.
4. Individual Prevention Strategies: Learning about Anger (*Learning about Anger, Handout 2.1*)
    - Identifying anger.
    - Slowed breathing techniques.
5. Dyadic Intervention Strategy: Time-Out (*Steps to an Effective Time-Out, Handout 2.2*)
    - Teach and provide rationale for time-out.
    - In-session practice of the technique.
6. Out-of-Session Assignments (Handout 2.3)
    - *Learning about Anger (Handout 2.1)*
    - *Steps to an Effective Time-Out (Handout 2.2)*
    - *You've Been Caught Doing Something Nice (Handout 2.3)*
7. Check-Out

*Administer the patient and partner versions of PCL/relationship happiness.

## Review of Out-of-Session Assignments

One small but powerful tip in managing and pacing sessions in CBCT for PTSD is to begin each session subsequent to the first session with the question "How did the out-of-session practice go?" Social convention and some therapy models would lead you as a therapist to ask a more open-ended question such as "How are things going?" For many couples, this will open up the dialogue to discuss myriad topics, and before you know it you are engaged in problem solving or crisis management and 20 or more minutes of the session have passed. Issues of potential self- or other-harm are certainly reasons to put off the content of the session. All other topics should optimally be woven into the material being presented at a given session (e.g., used as material for practicing communication skills).

Ask the couple what they took away from reviewing the *Cycle of PTSD Symptoms and Recovery from Trauma* (Handout 1.2) and reading the *Trauma and Relationships* (Handout 1.4) outside of session. Ask what questions they might have about these handouts.

Next, review the couple's completion of the OOSA *You've Been Caught Doing Something Nice* (Handout 1.6). Couples will often comment on the amount of positive behaviors in their relationship previously overlooked (i.e., selective attention). If they don't, orient them to this. Reinforce the importance of staying aware of positive behaviors in their relationship as negative aspects are being addressed in the course of therapy. This strategy can also be used with other family members, such as the couple's children, to increase positivity, enhance emotional engagement, and decrease avoidance.

Finally, review each partner's responses to the *Trauma Impact Questions–I* (TIQ-I; Handout 1.5). Have each member of the couple read what he or she wrote in response to the questions, with each partner sharing his or her answer to each question before proceeding to the next. In reviewing the questions, it is important to keep the following principles in mind:

- Note first the similarities in their responses to each of the questions (i.e., impact on relationship, ways of making sense of traumatic events, and thoughts in each of the areas) to reinforce their shared understanding of how PTSD has impacted their relationship, how they view the traumatic event(s), and their shared worldview in each of the content areas.
- **Gently** point out the differences in each member's responses. Here you are planting seeds for the work to follow and reinforcing the tolerance of individual differences in their relationship.
- Notice the ways that PTSD has limited their relationship and the ways in which their respective thoughts and beliefs are keeping them stuck in PTSD and relationship problems. These are the stuck points that you will subsequently prioritize to be targeted in the therapy.

**Note: Take the TIQ-I (*Handout 1.5*) completed by each partner and keep them for review in Phase 3 of the therapy and at the final session. Indicate to the couple that they will be completing a similar worksheet at the end of therapy to mark changes in the impact of trauma**

**(not necessarily PTSD) on their relationship and ways that they perceive themselves, traumatic experiences, and their relationship.**

Each individual's response to the TIQ-I should be used to formulate (1) the ways that PTSD has impacted and is maintained in their relationship and (2) stuck points in each partner's thinking that are maintaining PTSD and relationship discord. It is important to note that although CBCT for PTSD is a manualized therapy, the therapist must use his or her clinical skills to conceptualize the factors maintaining PTSD and relationship problems. The TIQ-I is designed to heighten motivation by increasing the couple's awareness of how PTSD is impacting each of them as individuals and their relationship. It is also designed to give the therapist a head start in understanding the role of PTSD in the couple's relationship and the cognitive factors at work that are maintaining the individual- and couple-level problems.

Figure 2.1 provides a sample TIQ-I completed by Susan and Jake, described in Chapter 2. There is substantial information for case conceputalization gleaned from the relatively brief answers provided by the couple. In this example, the effect of Susan's emotional numbing on the relationship is apparent based on each of their responses to the first question. She has also provided several places and situations that she avoids that the therapist can be sure are added to the approach list. Her reexperiencing symptoms in the form of nightmares have caused the couple to sleep separately, and her hyperarousal-related hypervigilance has contributed to Susan's desire to sleep on the couch, specifically because her back is "against something and not vulnerable." In addition, Jake's accommodation of Susan's symptoms by avoiding disclosure of times that he is upset by her is revealed. Susan's responses to the second question reveals her problematic appraisals related to her sexual assault; specifically, she is engaging in hindsight bias and undoing (described in Session 9) by thinking that she should not have gone back to the perpetrator's apartment and that she "should have noticed that [the perpetrator] was suspicious looking." She evidences happily-ever-after thinking in noting that if she had fought back, there would have only been good outcomes. Jake's response to the second question seems to imply that he blames Susan for her sexual assault, given his comments that "we stand to learn something from them" and "so Susan needs to learn or change something in her life." He has also introduced the notion of religion or spirituality in making sense of the trauma, and this provides the therapist with early indication that it will be important to factor in these beliefs in how each of them construe the event.

Susan's and Jake's responses to the core areas (i.e., trust, control, emotional closeness, physical closeness) provide information not only about their individual beliefs for each, but also how their individual beliefs are likely to interact with one another. Susan does not trust herself or others, and Jake seems to share some concerns about his ability to trust Susan in some situations. It would be wise for the therapist to determine the nature of the situations in which Jake has some distrust of Susan to enrich his case conceptualization. Otherwise, Jake seems to have reasonably balanced views about trust, which are likely to be an asset in the therapy. Both are struggling with thoughts of being out of control in their relationship, and it seems as though emotional volatility contributes to these beliefs. Both recognize the emotional distance in the relationship, and Susan's emotional distance seems generalized beyond her relationship with Jake. Susan's "repulsion" of being touched and feelings of disgust (seemingly about sexuality, although the generalizability of this disgust to all types of physical touch should be queried) seem to have contributed to frustration and conflict over the physical aspects of their relationship.

Name: *SUSAN*

1. **How has trauma or PTSD affected our relationship to date? How has it impacted my thoughts, feelings, and behaviors about our relationship?**

   *I've shut down. I just don't want to deal with it or anything for that matter. Jake complains about this. I often think that people are out to get me—especially men. I don't like to be out at night or near bus shelters in the night or day. We don't sleep in the same bed because I often wake him up in the night thrashing around in bed. I also like sleeping on the couch because my back is against something and not vulnerable.*

2. **Why did the traumatic event(s) happen to me or my partner?**

   *I shouldn't have gone back to his apartment after going out, and especially after drinking. I wasn't drunk, but I wasn't as alert as I should have been. The guy was just a pervert, and I should have noticed that he was suspicious looking. I didn't fight back, which I regret, because it might have caused someone else to hear what was going on or for him to stop.*

3. **What do I believe in each of the following areas, as it relates to *me, my partner, and others*?**

   **Trust:**

   *don't trust myself anymore. I also don't entirely trust Jake. I don't trust anyone, but especially men.*

   **Control:**

   *I feel like I'm completely out of control of myself and my relationship with Jake. It feels like I'm on a roller coaster of emotions. It is so bad that I can't do work. I used to be so capable and now I'm a mess. I have no control over others.*

   **Emotional Closeness:**

   *I don't know how this applies to myself. Jake and I seem close at times, but at others times we are miles apart. When we start to get close, I wind up lashing out at him. I'm not close to my family or many friends. I do have one friend, Ashley, whom I'm close to, but no one else really.*

   **Physical Closeness:**

   *I don't know how this applies to myself really. We have not had sex in 2 years. I can't stand being touched—it repulses me. This frustrates Jake and I understand that, but it feels disgusting.*

   *(cont.)*

**FIGURE 2.1.** Susan's and Jake's Trauma Impact Questions–I.

Name: _JAKE_

1. **How has trauma or PTSD affected our relationship to date? How has it impacted my thoughts, feelings, and behaviors about our relationship?**

   *It has (at times) kept Susan emotionally closed off. I have adjusted to not always telling her when she has upset me to avoid upsetting her. We rarely share a bed because of her nightmares, and she can't stand someone being close to her when she is in bed. Some days I feel like I've lost her to what happened.*

2. **Why did the traumatic event(s) happen to me or my partner?**

   *I feel like these things happened because we stand to learn something from them. God has set plans for each of us, so Susan needs to learn or change something in her life.*

3. **What do I believe in each of the following areas, as it relates to *me, my partner, and others*?**

   **Trust:**

   *I generally trust my judgment and instincts. I trust Susan in most situations without me there, but in others, I stress the whole time, because she gets easily upset. There are some bad people in the world who will take advantage of others, but I think most people in my life are trustworthy.*

   **Control:**

   *I feel like I'm pretty in control of myself, but I often feel out of control of our relationship. I feel like Susan tries to control me at times because of what happened to her. Sometimes my boss is controlling, but I'm not easily controlled.*

   **Emotional Closeness:**

   *Susan and I are sometimes close, but then I feel like she pushes me away. It feels like there is a wall between us, and I don't know how to break through it. I have some close friends and I'm close to my family.*

   **Physical Closeness:**

   *Susan and I enjoyed being physically intimate early on in our relationship, but that has died off. We rarely even hold hands. She doesn't like to be touched unless it is on her terms and that is very frustrating. People consider me to be a touchy [physically demonstrative] guy.*

**FIGURE 2.1.** *(cont.)*

***IMPORTANT NOTE:*** If the couple did not complete the assignments, it is crucial that this be addressed immediately. It is helpful to explore the role of avoidance in completing assignments, methods to overcoming other barriers to completing the assignments (e.g., scheduling times to complete them, alternating responsibility between the two of them for making sure the assignments are completed), and revisiting the rationale for the OOSAs. Moreover, any assignment not completed outside of session should be added to the next OOSA schedule. It is especially important in these early sessions to establish the importance of OOSAs. In our experience, clinicians can sometimes be reluctant to address OOSA adherence directly, reporting that they believe that they are shaming or chastising the couple. It is important to keep in mind that without this outside work, the couple will not be receiving an adequate dose of therapy. For the couple's benefit, and the benefit of each individual suffering from PTSD or another mental health condition, we strongly recommend that you intervene as nonjudgmentally and in as matter-of-fact a manner as possible, stressing the important benefits of the OOSAs for the couple and for each partner individually.

As discussed earlier, we recommend that you revisit the treatment contract and the couple's commitment to therapy if two sessions' worth of OOSAs have not been completed (i.e., at Session 3 they have not completed an adequate number of OOSAs, approximately 75% of the assignments). In proceeding further without some level of OOSA adherence, you are offering a treatment experience that may have compromised effectiveness or may even be ineffective, leading to perceived inadequate treatment (or worse yet treatment failure).

## Trauma Focus and Disclosure

Because of your thorough pretreatment assessment, you will know about the index event leading to the PTSD diagnosis before you start the protocol. It is important to bear in mind that the partner may not know much, if anything, about the details of the index traumatic event, or may know that the traumatized partner has experienced multiple events and is not sure which index event will be the initial focus of treatment. The level of partner knowledge about the traumatic event(s) will likely be evident in the course of discussions but also in reviewing the TIQ-I (i.e., a partner responds that she does not have any appraisals because she does not know about the traumatic events). Thus, there should be a brief discussion to clarify that the couple and the therapist are in agreement about the index event (or events in the case of a dual-PTSD couple). You should then explain why the index traumatic event is identified in the therapy. More specifically, the couple should be educated that the most distressing event is chosen as the first focus of treatment because of the likelihood of gains surrounding that event generalizing to the other traumatic events. The couple should be clear that you expect improvements related to other traumatic events, but any events not seemingly improved by an initial and successful focus on the index event can be directly addressed in therapy later.

It is important that you have an up-front discussion with the couple about the **disclosure of specific traumatic material and the expectations surrounding it**. You should be clear with the couple that they are not expected to immerse themselves in specific details about their traumas because the treatment is not an "exposure" treatment per se. However, there will inevitably be some trauma details shared to put the experiences back into their proper context. Clients are encouraged to talk about their trauma history with their loved ones, but are discouraged from providing in-depth, gory, and/or gratuitous retellings of their experiences.

Encourage the traumatized individuals to focus on the emotions surrounding their memories and the meaning of those events for the here and now versus an explicit retelling of the details of their traumatic experience. We often tell couples that we will be discussing the event as if from a "10,000-foot view." It is helpful to inform clients that the goal is not to forget memories but rather to decrease the distress attached to them and to make more sense of their experiences. Thus, relaying the specific details is less important than fully experiencing and expressing the emotions attached to them.

It is important to consider the fear clients may have about working on their traumatic material. Frequent concerns include:

1. Partner's ability to handle the information (e.g., partner will "freak out" or "break down").
2. Increase in symptoms as a result of talking about the trauma (e.g., fears about flashbacks).
3. Changes in the relationship because of disclosure (e.g., partner might judge them or leave because of the knowledge).
4. Level of detail to provide to others.

Partners may also have concerns about the traumatized individual's disclosure of trauma-related material. For example, the partner may fear that in discussing the traumatic event, the traumatized partner will become very angry or otherwise emotionally dysregulated and that this will, in turn, disturb whatever equilibrium they have established in their relationship.

It is important for you to gauge each partner's desires and/or concerns about hearing trauma-related information. It is our experience that traumatized individuals often underestimate their loved one's interest and ability to handle their disclosures. However, you should carefully anticipate the partner's reactions to these disclosures and facilitate a safe context for the couple to communicate about this material. Bear in mind that both members of the couple may have traumatic material to disclose. Material that may be particularly distressing for clients includes information about atrocities, sexual victimization, and violence against civilians during war. It is important to keep in mind that disclosure can be threatening or difficult for others to hear because of their own feelings of vulnerability, powerlessness, or helplessness that such disclosures can engender. Normalize such reactions but, especially as therapy progresses, challenge the notion that avoidance of such disclosures will bring greater "safety" to the traumatized partner and relationship.

*As I mentioned previously, we will consider how trauma has impacted your relationship and each of your thoughts, feelings, and behaviors. It is important for us to have a brief conversation about the trauma that we will be working on (or working on first if there have been multiple traumas). We want to choose the most distressing trauma to work on first because improvements related to that trauma will improve your symptoms related to other traumas that have been experienced. If, however, we have success with working on that trauma and symptoms related to other traumas have not improved, we can work on those other traumas. According to the assessment results, [PTSD+ partner], you identified _____ (e.g., sexual assault by a prior boyfriend, motor vehicle accident, combat trauma) as the most distressing trauma. Is that correct? [If dual PTSD, confirm understanding of index trauma for both individuals.]*

*We will not be covering explicit details of traumatic experiences. This is not an "exposure therapy," in which either of you will be asked to go over and over the traumatic memories until you are less distressed about them. However, understanding how you have made meaning of the traumatic event(s) directly influences how well you have recovered from that event(s). It also influences how you think about yourself and your partner in your relationship and, consequently, how you feel about one another. Thus, this phase of therapy in particular will involve some conversation about the traumatic event(s) in order to understand how you make meaning of the traumatic event(s) you have experienced. In terms of level of detail, we will be discussing the event as if from a 10,000-foot view. It is a more distanced approach to addressing the trauma memories.*

*Disclosure of traumatic events to a trusted, supportive other improves recovery from the traumatic events. Therefore, there is reason to believe that sharing traumatic events in a safe and supportive environment is therapeutic in and of itself. There are several important ingredients that both of you bring to the recipe for successful disclosure and discussion of how trauma has impacted you and your relationship. Most generally, there has to be a willingness for both of you to approach and share the traumatic memories, respond supportively to one another, and be willing to consider different ways of making sense of the experiences. My role will be to make this very important work as safe and positive as possible for the two of you.*

*In order for me to get an idea of your possible concerns and past experiences with trauma disclosure [sample questions follow; all questions do not need to be asked]:*

*How much have each of you talked about what happened to _____?*
*What concerns do each of you have about sharing traumatic material?*
*What do you imagine will happen when we talk about the trauma(s)?*
*Have you had prior negative experiences when you've shared your traumatic event(s)?*
*Are there things that I can do to make this aspect of our work as positive as possible?*

## Addressing Negative Behaviors as Barriers to Safety

Couple research is clear that negative behaviors have a relatively greater effect on relationship satisfaction than do positive behaviors (Gottman & Levenson, 1992). Thus, an early emphasis is placed on decreasing very negative behaviors in the relationship.

There are six key concepts in providing psychoeducation to the couple regarding why these negative behaviors are addressed early and directly in the therapy.

1. **Conflict is inevitable in ALL relationships.** The goal of this therapy is not to have the couple stop arguing but rather to help them argue *more effectively* (i.e., more kindly and respectfully).
2. There are **negative behaviors that have particularly potent negative effects** on relationships, and these behaviors need to be decreased to improve the safety in their relationship. It is crucial that **hostility and contempt** be decreased in order for partners to feel safe with one another. You can differentiate nonhostile criticism that focuses on a particular behavior (e.g., "I don't like it when you leave your socks on the floor") from hostility or contempt that serves as a negative characterological attribution and global rejection of the person ("You're a jerk!" "You're a lazy, good-for-nothing").
3. Specific to PTSD, **increased irritability and anger** are part and parcel of the hyperarousal symptoms of PTSD. Persons with PTSD consistently perceive more **threat** in their social environment. This psychoeducation is not to condone anger expression in the couple's relationship. Rather, it is designed to point out the role that the disorder has in generating conflict and how the couple handles that conflict. Remind the couple of the fight-or-flight physiological reaction and how it continues to linger and "misfire" in the case of PTSD. Note that this session is designed to help **manage the "fight" part of that reaction.**
4. Related to the third principle, relationships in which a partner has PTSD are at risk for **a range of aggressive behaviors.**
5. Individuals with PTSD are at risk for substance abuse, and **substance use synergistically increases the risk for relationship conflict and aggression in those with PTSD.**
6. Finally, those who have been traumatized were not safe at the time of the event. Our goal is to **increase the amount of safety** that they and their loved one can experience in their intimate relationship in order to facilitate recovery.

Be very direct, yet compassionate, in educating the couple on the deleterious effects of **very negative** relationship behaviors, such as **verbal, physical, or sexual abuse; threats to leave the relationship; and ongoing infidelity.** As discussed in Part I, all couples should be screened for a wide spectrum of physically aggressive behaviors that they may have perpetrated or been the victim of over the course of their relationship. Couples in which severe abuse is currently of issue should be excluded from therapy, and treatment specific to this behavior should be the first priority. If more severe levels of aggression are shared in the therapy, safety planning and direct targeting of this behavior should be the focus of treatment before proceeding with a course of CBCT for PTSD.

All of these negative behaviors should be inquired about and discussed as nonjudgmentally as possible without condoning their continuation. Clearly assist the couple in understanding that engaging in or tolerating very negative behaviors in the relationship may promote a cycle of individual feelings of anxiety and shame and a decrease in safety. Challenging this cycle provides opportunities to build a more positive, safe connection to one another while lowering their distress. It may be tempting to collude with the couple by resisting specific and clear discussions of these topics. The process of challenging their avoidance and building safety assists in deepening the couple's alliance while simultaneously freeing them to move toward other feared affect, situations, or topics. To facilitate this discussion and a couple-level understanding of how a series of negative behaviors unfolded and ultimately culminated in verbal or physical aggression, it can be helpful for the therapist to say nonjudgmentally, "Help me understand what happens between the two of you when one or both of you are angry."

## Individual Prevention Strategies: Learning about Anger

The primary prevention strategies against negative behavior during this phase of CBCT for PTSD to be taught to the couple are self-awareness of their own anger and distressing feelings and slowed breathing. Many people, especially those with PTSD, do not recognize early signs of anger or their cognitions that fuel their anger. To facilitate this self-awareness, engage the couple in a discussion about **the bodily sensations, cognitions, and behaviors** that accompany their feelings of anger. Have partners observe in themselves and each other what they experience when they are angry. Orient the couple to *Learning About Anger* (*Handout 2.1*), which you will ask them to complete for their OOSA later.

### *Identifying Anger*

Specifically discuss the **earliest signs of anger** that the partners notice. This is an important goal of the prevention strategy. By increasing their awareness of the earliest signs of their anger, they can then make choices about how to keep their anger at an optimal level to facilitate their own personal health and the health of their relationship. The goal is not to eliminate anger but rather to keep it at a level at which they can behave most effectively. Emphasize that anger is an important emotion. It alerts us to when we *might* have been wronged (emphasis is added to convey the possibility that our perceptions of wrongdoing on the part of another may be incorrect if more information is gathered).

One disorder-specific point of psychoeducation about anger to impart is the distinction between emotions that emanate from **perceived threat versus wrongdoing**. This is a subtle but important distinction that may be helpful for the couple, particularly the PTSD+ partner, in discriminating emotion states further. Remind the couple that PTSD causes people to walk around on high alert, scanning for perceived threat in the environment. One option for reacting to threat perceived in the environment is to fight. The other option is to avoid (flight). Avoidance is usually more readily associated with fear. It is tempting to confuse the fight instinct and associated behavior with feelings of anger when it is really fueled by fear of something perceived to be hurtful in the environment.

Bear in mind that some couples with a PTSD+ partner manage conflict through **reactive or chronic avoidance**. In other words, they avoid immediately in reaction to negative affect experienced in the relationship or they have developed a pattern of chronic disengagement from one another to avoid the possibility of experiencing more negative emotions or behaviors in their relationship. The overarching goal for these couples is to encourage reengagement with one another about their conflict, exploring their fears about what would happen if there was greater sharing about their areas of conflict. There are often fears that someone might "blow up," say things that he or she might regret, or cause the destruction of the relationship. It is also important in motivating them for reengagement to inquire what they are missing out on in their relationship as a result of their chronic disengagement.

## Slowed Breathing and Other Individual Strategies for Anger/Affect Management

Brainstorm with the couple strategies that each of them use to manage their anger. The one intervention that seems to have nearly universal helpfulness in managing distressing emotions in general is slowed breathing. Increased respiration is one of the cardinal signs of engagement of the fight-or-flight system and general arousal. Slowed respiration can soothe or back off that system when it misfires or when one is distressed.

We encourage you to briefly practice slowed breathing with the couple in session to illustrate how to do it and to demonstrate its effects. Specifically, ask the partners to place their hands comfortably on the arms of a chair or on their lap and then practice inhaling for two counts and exhaling for four counts. Ask that they do **at least** three rounds of inhaling–exhaling—and more if needed—to alleviate distress.

*One strategy for managing anger and other distressing emotions that is generally helpful to almost everyone is to slow down one's breathing. When you are upset or your fight-or-flight system has been activated, your respiration increases to pump blood throughout your system and mobilize you for action. You can counteract and soothe that system by slowing down your breathing. The exhalation of breath, in particular, slows the system. So we recommend that you inhale for two counts and then exhale for four counts. Let me illustrate. [Breathe in for 2 seconds and out for 4 seconds.]*

*Let's practice the breathing together. You can even close your eyes if you are comfortable and if that calms you down further. Place your hands comfortably on the arms of the chair or in your lap and then [pattern] inhale for 1, 2; exhale for 1, 2, 3, 4; inhale for 1, 2; exhale for 1, 2, 3, 4. . . .*

*How does the breathing make you feel? Do you feel calmer?*

*It is helpful to do **at least** three inhale–exhale cycles, although many people find more cycles helpful.*

In a minority of cases, slowed breathing may increase distress, especially in those with a history of panic attacks. In those cases, inquire whether there are other strategies that have helped manage distress. It is not imperative that slowed breathing be used.

## Dyadic Intervention Strategy: Time-Out

Provide the couple with *Steps to an Effective Time-Out* (Handout 2.2). Review each of the steps (STOP) carefully, highlighting several notions:

- **S = SELF.** Time-out is *not a punitive measure* to use against your partner. Time-out is an early intervention technique. It is a mutually agreed-upon technique for the couple to use to deescalate situations and to prevent saying or doing things they might later regret. They are not timing *each other* out. Rather, time-outs are for them as individuals. They are to be used to become more aware of distress levels and to maintain enough emotional control to communicate effectively. A good analogy to use is that of a sports team calling a time-out to regroup and determine what plays they are going to execute when the clock resumes. Encourage clients to *notice their own varying levels of anger or other distress*. As mentioned previously, clients are likely to tell you that they go from 0 to 10 (10 = rage) in their anger in seconds. Clients should consider how angry they generally are and how far (or not so far) they have to go before they become enraged.

- **T = TIME-OUT.** Some couples have named the technique something other than time-out (e.g., "pause time," "break time," "downtime") to avoid any connotations of punishment. Encourage the couple to use a mutually agreed-upon label that works for them. The couple should agree on both a *nonverbal* and a *verbal* indication of the time-out period. At the point of calling a time-out, the couple commits to stopping their communication immediately (no taunting or continued discussion). They also agree on an *amount of time and circumstance* for resuming their communication. In this vein, encourage the couple to go no longer than *30 minutes* before checking back in with one another at the predetermined meeting place, if only to request more time for the time-out. Multiple 30-minute check-ins may be necessary before communication can resume. This is very helpful for minimizing any demand–withdraw pattern that may be occurring.
- **O = OUTLET.** While taking a time-out, partners are encouraged to use their outlet as a time to soothe themselves. Therefore, we encourage slowed breathing and avoidance of activities that might fuel their negative emotions (e.g., punching on a punching bag, ruminating on the partner's wrongdoing). During the outlet time, the couple is encouraged to clarify for themselves what one or two things are most upsetting and to identify one thing that they might do to facilitate the communication.
- **P = PROCESS.** The final step is for the couple to return to the agreed-upon place to resume the process of discussing the topic that resulted in a time-out. Upon returning, the couple is urged to focus on what they can do to improve their communication.

There are several key notions in making time-outs effective for those couples in which at least one partner has PTSD:

1. It is *key* that the couple *returns to communicate*. Couples with a PTSD+ partner might tell you that they use time-outs all of the time. In fact, they AVOID, never returning to the previously conflictual situation for further resolution. This tends to be a very typical characteristic of couples in which one or more partners have PTSD. Watch out for this tendency. **Stress that the value of time-out is only as good as there is time-in.**
2. Remind the couple that they may not have *full resolution* of the issue that necessitated a time-out. Rather, the goal is to get *more* resolution and to use better skills that lead to less relationship damage. It is helpful to remind them that the goal is not to get rid of disagreements—this is an inevitable part of interpersonal relationships—but rather to improve how they handle those disagreements.
3. It is important to point out that time-outs work best in a *feedback loop* fashion. If a time-out is called and they return to the situation only to escalate again, another time-out can be called. They can return to the situation for another time-out and so on. After you have gone over the steps to an effective time-out, **have each member of the couple**

**practice calling a time-out in session.** Ask the couple to consider and describe a recent conflict. Have them imagine it escalating to the point of needing to call a time-out. Then ask the couple to go through the time-out steps, with each person practicing calling a time-out. This is the first of many opportunities for the couple to practice the skills in session while you observe and coach. It is important that each of them have this initial experience of calling a time-out in session to increase the likelihood that they will do it out of session.

To facilitate a more realistic version of the couple's time-out practice, ask the couple to turn their chairs to face one another. This will decrease the possibility that they will speak to you versus one another. Also, note that you will be observing or "eavesdropping" on their communication to facilitate or "coach" them in learning the skills. Normalize that it might feel artificial or awkward to practice these skills in session but that it is important for them to have the experience of initially doing it with someone around to help them. **The couple will be much more likely to do the technique outside of session if they have had the experience of walking through the steps in session.**

Actively make corrections and provide feedback about each partner's practice in as supportive and nonjudgmental a manner as possible. In this and future sessions, you may need to role-model skills for the couple to understand and learn them. Remember to simultaneously provide positive reinforcement for specific aspects of the skills that they are doing well.

## Out-of-Session Assignments

Orient the couple to the *OOSA summary* (*Handout 2.3*) for this session and point out the following assignments:

- Request that each member of the couple self-monitor at least one episode of anger or distress prior to the next session, using *Learning about Anger* (*Handout 2.1*). The anger does not need to be in response to the partner. Also, ask them to write about the earliest signs that they observe of their partner's anger. These observations can come from an instance between now and the next session or prior instances. Go over the worksheet and make sure that they understand what they are being asked to do.
- Request that each member of the couple call at least one time-out over the course of the week and complete the section of *Steps to an Effective Time-Out* (*Handout 2.2*) related to their calling a time-out. Inform them that a major fight should *not* be initiated in order to practice the technique. In fact, a minor argument is more effective for learning the technique because they are less distressed. If there are no disagreements at all, they should each walk through the steps of time-out together.
- Ask the couple to monitor daily for positive behaviors that they catch each other doing between now and the next session (*Handout 2.3*). Fine-tune any use of this intervention to maximize its effects. For example, did they actually do it on a daily basis? Did they point out the positive behavior verbally to their partner? Is the form placed somewhere that is obvious and accessible for the two of them?

## Check-Out

Ask the couple how the session was for each of them. Are there any lingering concerns or questions? Infuse hopefulness and predict success in completing the OOSAs as they leave the session.

## HANDOUT 2.1

# Learning about Anger

Name: _____

---

**Situation about which I was angry:**
_____

**What were the earliest signs that I was angry?**
_____
_____
_____
_____
_____

**What did I do to increase or decrease my anger (e.g., breathing)?**
_____
_____
_____
_____
_____
_____

---

**MY PARTNER'S ANGER**

**What are the earliest signs that my partner is angry?**
_____
_____
_____
_____
_____

---

From *Cognitive-Behavioral Conjoint Therapy for PTSD: Harnessing the Healing Power of Relationships* by Candice M. Monson and Steffany J. Fredman. Copyright 2012 by The Guilford Press. Permission to photocopy this handout is granted to purchasers of this book for personal use only (see copyright page for details).

HANDOUT 2.2

# Steps to an Effective Time-Out

S = *Self*
1. What is the level of your own distress?
   (0 = none → 10 = as intense as you can imagine)
   5–6 = yellow light
   7–8 = red light
2. Time-outs are for your sake.

T = *Time-Out*
1. Nonverbal and verbal indication.
2. Immediate stop in communication.
3. Agree on an amount of time and circumstance for returning.

O = *Outlet*
1. BREATHE.
2. Avoid activities that fuel your negative emotions.
3. Clarify what one or two things are most upsetting.
4. Consider one thing you can do to improve communication.

P = *Process*
1. Return at the agreed-upon time and circumstance.
2. Resume communication, with focus on your goal for improvement. REMEMBER: TIME-OUT IS ONLY AS GOOD AS TIME-IN.
3. Self-monitor.

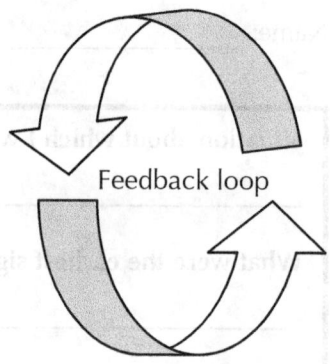

Feedback loop

| Time-Out Caller | Circumstances | What Worked | Areas to Improve |
|---|---|---|---|
| Sherry | We were fighting over how we spend our money. I did not want Tom to buy more clothes. | • Stopped fighting when time-out was called.<br>• We came back at the time we agreed upon.<br>• We called a second time-out. | • We developed "ammunition" while we were apart.<br>• We didn't focus on improving our own communication. |
|  |  |  |  |
|  |  |  |  |

From *Cognitive-Behavioral Conjoint Therapy for PTSD: Harnessing the Healing Power of Relationships* by Candice M. Monson and Steffany J. Fredman. Copyright 2012 by The Guilford Press. Permission to photocopy this handout is granted to purchasers of this book for personal use only (see copyright page for details).

HANDOUT 2.3

# Out-of-Session Assignments
## Session 2. Safety Building

1. Each of you should complete the worksheet *Learning about Anger* (*Handout 2.1*). The top part of the sheet asks each of you to describe an episode of anger that you experienced during the week prior to the next session. Note: Your partner **does not** need to be the focus of your anger. The bottom portion asks you to write about early signs of your partner's anger. These signs can come from an instance between now and the next session or prior instances that you have observed.

2. Before our next session, **each** of you should practice calling a time-out. Do **not** provoke a major argument to practice the time-out technique. In fact, smaller disagreements are better for developing the skill to use in larger disagreements. During both time-outs, practice the slowed breathing that you did in today's session.

    Write about each of the time-outs on the *Steps to an Effective Time-Out* (*Handout 2.2*). Report who called the time-out and the circumstances under which the time-out was called. Also, include what was good about the time-out and what could be improved for future time-outs.

3. Continue noticing the positive aspects of your relationship by completing the *You've Been Caught Doing Something Nice* form below. Place it somewhere noticeable for the two of you to complete on a daily basis.

**Next appointment:** _____ @ _____.

### YOU'VE BEEN CAUGHT DOING SOMETHING NICE

Week of: _____

|  | *Person Caught:* _____ | *Person Caught:* _____ |
|---|---|---|
| *Sunday* | | |
| *Monday* | | |
| *Tuesday* | | |
| *Wednesday* | | |
| *Thursday* | | |
| *Friday* | | |
| *Saturday* | | |

---

From *Cognitive-Behavioral Conjoint Therapy for PTSD: Harnessing the Healing Power of Relationships* by Candice M. Monson and Steffany J. Fredman. Copyright 2012 by The Guilford Press. Permission to photocopy this handout is granted to purchasers of this book for personal use only (see copyright page for details).

**PHASE 2**

# Satisfaction Enhancement and Undermining Avoidance

# SESSION 3

# Listening and Approaching

---

### SUMMARY OF SESSION CONTENT

#### Goals

- Provide a strong foundation for understanding the role of avoidance in PTSD and relationship problems.
- Introduce communication skills building as a method of decreasing conflict and increasing positive exchanges between the partners.
- Normalize the possible exacerbation of symptoms as signs that the couple is engaged in the therapy and noticing symptoms of PTSD rather than avoiding.
- Teach the skill of paraphrasing.

#### Key Interventions

1. Review of Out-of-Session Assignments
   - *Learning about Anger* (Handout 2.1)
   - *Steps to an Effective Time-Out* (Handout 2.2)
   - *You've Been Caught Doing Something Nice* (Handout 2.3)
2. Psychoeducation about PTSD, Avoidance, and Intimate Relationship Functioning *(PTSD and Avoidance, Handout 3.1)*
   - Operant conditioning.
   - Avoidance of feelings, thoughts, and memories.
   - Experiential avoidance and intimate relationship satisfaction.
3. Introduction to Communication Skills Training
   - Psychoeducation about the importance of communication skills.
   - Describe the three communication skills areas (listening/paraphrasing, sharing thoughts and feelings, problem solving/decision making).
4. Effective Listening Skills
   - Provide rationale for paraphrasing.
   - Teach paraphrasing to the couple.
   - In-session practice of paraphrasing.
5. Out-of-Session Assignments (Handout 3.3)
   - *Notice Positive Behaviors in Each Other*
   - *PTSD and Avoidance* (Handout 3.1)
   - *Avoidance List* (Handout 3.2)
   - *Catch Each Other Paraphrasing* (Handout 3.3)
6. Check-Out

*Administer the patient and partner versions of PCL/relationship happiness.

## Review of Out-of-Session Assignments

### *Learning about Anger (Handout 2.1)*

Have each member of the couple review their responses to the worksheet. While they are reviewing their responses, listen for themes in a given partner's thinking and behavioral responses. Also, emphasize early recognition of anger signs and any strategies that were helpful or not helpful in managing anger at an optimal level (e.g., slowed breathing). Brainstorm possible other strategies that may be helpful in managing anger at that optimal level. Encourage each partner to reflect on what new information he or she learned about the other.

### *Steps to an Effective Time-Out (Handout 2.2)*

The couple may indicate that the time-out steps felt stilted, awkward, or unnatural. Validate this experience: "Of course it felt awkward, because it is a completely new way of interacting with one another." Confirm that each member of the couple used *all* four steps to an effective time-out (STOP). Watch for the possibility that the couple did not return to the topic for further resolution (i.e., time-in). Remember that time-out can be used as a method of avoidance. Thus, check carefully that the couple returned to the topic for which one of them called a time-out.

If they did not successfully use the time-out steps, brainstorm and troubleshoot how they might use the time-out procedures more effectively in the future. We have found that a number of couples come to this session indicating that they had nothing about which to call a time-out. This is especially true for couples experiencing early improvements in the therapy and highly avoidant couples. We remind them that even minor episodes of irritation (expected in any relationship) can be used for time-outs. We reiterate that these minor topics and levels of distress are great training ground for the time-out procedures. If the couple did not complete the assignment, review the steps in session and ask them to demonstrate the technique. Reassign the exercise for completion by next session.

### *You've Been Caught Doing Something Nice (Handout 2.3)*

Review this worksheet and highlight the positivity that is occurring between the partners. Solicit their own reactions about this positivity, noting the tendency for negativity to override attention to the positivity in their relationship. Point out that although you will not be asking them to continue to write down positive behaviors on a daily basis, in subsequent sessions you will be inquiring about examples of positive behavior that they have noticed in their partner.

## Psychoeducation about PTSD, Avoidance, and Intimate Relationship Functioning

Point out to the couple that they have successfully completed the first phase of the therapy, focused on understanding PTSD and developing more safety in their relationship. They are now beginning Phase 2 of the therapy, focused on overcoming avoidance and enhancing their relationship through improved communication.

It is important that the couple understands that avoidance and emotional numbing are key culprits in maintaining PTSD. You should provide psychoeducation that one of the predominant emotions involved in PTSD is anxiety. At a simplistic level, individuals with PTSD have become "phobic," or afraid of the memories and emotions associated with their traumatic experiences as well as reminders that are associated with the traumatic experiences. In addition, traumatic experiences also involve other unpleasant emotions that people *choose* to avoid. These emotions include, but are not limited to, guilt, shame, horror, disgust, anger, helplessness, sadness, and grief. Fear of the memory and trauma-related reminders is likely to be obvious to the client and his or her partner. However, they may be less familiar with (1) the generalization of this fear to include the experience of emotions themselves and (2) the role of avoidance in maintaining PTSD symptoms and relationship problems.

*PTSD generally involves problems related to the emotion of fear. Other phobias, like fears of spiders, heights, or closed spaces, involve fear of situations or objects. In the case of PTSD, one's memory and reminders of the traumatic situation become feared.*

*In order to escape the painful emotions associated with those memories, traumatized individuals are likely to engage in a variety of methods of avoidance. This might mean avoidance of situations, places, people, smells, sights, temperatures, and so on that remind them of the traumatic situation.*

## *Operant Conditioning and Avoidance*

Orient the couple to *PTSD and Avoidance* (*Handout 3.1*) and remind them of the negatively reinforcing value of avoidance in relieving trauma-related distress. The graphic in the *PTSD and Avoidance* handout can also be used to underscore the reinforcing role of avoidance in PTSD.

*The upside of avoidance for all of us is that it relieves our anxiety or fear in the* **short** *run. Let's use your experiences as an example. [For example: if trauma memory relates to experiences in the military, one might feel anxiety or fear when hearing explosive sounds or when in hotter climates. If trauma involves a sexual assault, the client might feel anxiety or fear when he or she is around people of the same sex as the perpetrator, smells a certain cologne or perfume, engages in sexual activity, or goes to places similar to where the assault occurred.] Staying away from these trauma memory reminders alleviates your anxiety in the* **short** *run. However, avoidance catches up to us in the* **long** *run. Although it is a quick fix to our anxiety, it actually serves to increase our fears in the long run by reinforcing to us that we can't handle those situations. The longer and more frequently we avoid, the more we strengthen our fears.*

*This diagram [display the graphic in Handout 3.1] shows how avoidance and fear can spiral by feeding on each other. What situations, people, or feelings do either of you avoid that end up making the situation even worse?*

## Avoidance of Feelings, Thoughts, and Memories

It is important to emphasize to couples that avoidance can rear its ugly head in many forms beyond traditionally considered behavioral avoidance of trauma-related reminders. Individuals with PTSD and their intimate others can also become avoidant of emotional experiences more generally. A basic understanding of **experiential avoidance**, or the avoidance of private experiences such as feelings, memories, behavioral predispositions, or thoughts (Hayes & Gifford, 1997, for review), is presented to the couple. Unless the couple is fairly sophisticated, the term "experiential avoidance" should not be used. Rather, we describe it as a generalized and subtler form of avoidance: "fear of feeling."

Classic examples of avoidance beyond behavioral avoidance of trauma-related reminders outlined in the DSM nomenclature include the spectrum of compulsive behaviors (e.g., drugs, alcohol, smoking, sex, gambling, workaholism), self-injury, anger and aggression toward others, and dissociation. Suicidal ideation often serves as a form of emotional avoidance or escape from unpleasant circumstances and feelings. As a clinician, you want to be keenly observant of the various ways in which avoidance manifests in a given dyad and the ways in which the couple is accommodating such avoidance. The couple should also become sensitized to the ways in which they are colluding to avoid. These dyadic patterns will be specifically targeted beginning in this session.

*Avoidance is a slippery culprit. It can present itself in a variety of ways beyond just avoiding trauma-reminiscent situations, people, or things. Often, individuals with PTSD come to avoid their own internal experiences such as their thoughts, feelings, memories, and physical sensations. This tendency might be described as a "fear of feeling." Some common ways in which people avoid include substance abuse, obsessive thinking, overworking, emotional numbing, self-injury, fighting with others, eating, smoking, suicidal thoughts (e.g., escape), and injuring oneself.*

*How might you avoid individually or as a couple in these ways?[Solicit a few examples because the couple will communicate about this topic later in the session.]*

## Experiential Avoidance and Intimate Relationship Satisfaction

Expand on experiential avoidance as it relates to couples in particular, with a focus on emotions. In essence, avoiding one's emotions diminishes the expression of them, which, in turn, diminishes relationship satisfaction and intimacy.

*We know from research that emotions are the glue that holds relationships together. Couples who stay together and report the most satisfaction tell us that they share emotions with one another. A really important thing to know is that these emotions **don't** have to be only positive. It seems that the **sharing** of emotions is more important than the **type** of emotions shared, that is, whether the emotion shared is positive or negative.*

*Can you think of a time that your partner shared something with you and it made you feel closer to him or her? [If it was a negative experience or emotion, make sure to highlight that the **sharing** was more important than the fact that it may have been negative content or affect.]*

*Traumatized individuals and their loved ones often become emotionally avoidant or "emotionally phobic." They avoid emotional experiences and sharing their emotions with each other in their relationships. This is part of that more subtle avoidance that we discussed earlier. It is as though both members of the couple come to fear what might happen if they experience emotions in their relationship. This is a couple issue, not an individual issue, because it is rarely one person alone who avoids emotions. You might even fear the experience of positive emotions.*

# Introduction to Communication Skills Training

To transition to communication skills training, you should note to the couple that improved communication in their relationship serves (1) as an antidote to avoidance (i.e., approaching difficult and important conversations and feelings) and (2) to increase their relationship satisfaction.

**The following other points should be made in introducing communication skills training:**

1. Communication problems are the single most often reported problem among couples (Geiss & O'Leary, 1981), and improving communication is the single best prescription for improving relationship satisfaction.
2. Explain the importance of communication within relationships by describing how couples who are unable to express their ideas and feelings to each other are often excluded from each other's important experiences and decisions. They are left feeling disconnected from each other and their intimacy suffers.
3. Communication difficulties make serious conflict more likely when individuals are unable to have their needs met and resolve difficulties through communication with their partner.
4. These communication skills can be used across topics. If partners develop good skills, then they increase the likelihood of their being able to discuss all kinds of issues. The content is less relevant as their skills are honed.

**Points specific to couples in which one or both members have PTSD are as follows:**

1. Trauma-related symptoms may infringe on communication (e.g., dissociation, attention/concentration problems, irritability).
2. Behavioral and experiential avoidance can decrease the likelihood of communication with one another.

## *Communication Skills Areas*

Describe to the couple the three communication skill areas that will be developed in this phase of the therapy to help overcome their avoidance and increase their satisfaction:

1. Listening/paraphrasing.
2. Sharing thoughts and feelings.
3. Problem solving/decision making.

*In this phase of the therapy, we will be working on specific skills that will improve your communication with each other and help you overcome the avoidance that exists in your relationship. Today we will begin using* **listening skills***. These skills are the bedrock or foundation of good communication because it is difficult to respond effectively to someone if you haven't heard his or her message correctly. In other words, our first step is to make sure that a message sent was a message received.*

*Next, we will work on one channel of communication: sharing feelings and thoughts. We will work on this channel first because identifying how you think and feel and figuring out how you express those thoughts and feelings to someone is very important to effective communication. In the next session we'll focus on the feelings part of sharing thoughts and feelings, and then in the following session we will focus on the thoughts part. We will end this phase of therapy by focusing on how you solve problems and make decisions as a couple.*

*Improving these different skills will improve your communication, which will improve your relationship. These skills will also help defeat avoidance and consequently improve your PTSD symptoms. We will use these skills in the latter half of therapy to tackle the historical aspects of what keeps you stuck in PTSD and relationship problems.*

*What questions do you have about the communication skills?*

## Effective Listening Skills

You should stress to clients that listening is the foundation of all good communication. Thus, we begin with those skills. In introducing these skills, start with a discussion of instances in which they responded to their partner or someone else based on a misheard message. You will likely have examples from reviewing the pretreatment communication sample. The point to be made is that it is very difficult to respond effectively if you are responding to inaccurate (i.e., misperceived) information. It is also helpful to discuss instances in which they were preparing their next statement (i.e., rebuttal) versus listening to what another was saying.

An additional important concept to convey to the couple is the difference between **listening** and **hearing**. Hearing is the sensory act of receiving information auditorally (i.e., one has a hearing test, not a listening test). Listening encompasses much more information than just the words spoken by another. It includes paying attention to the "process" aspects of someone's message—their voice tone and inflection, feelings, nonverbals, and so on.

### *Paraphrasing*

The rationale when introducing the technique of paraphrasing is that paraphrasing is the best way to ensure that you *listened correctly* and has the benefit of containing affect around distressing topics by *slowing down communication.*

In this technique, couples are asked to take turns making statements and paraphrasing those statements. The couple should turn their chairs to face each other to make communication with one another (vs. the therapist) more conducive.

## Session 3. Listening and Approaching

- One member of the couple makes a statement(s) (**sending partner/speaker**).
- The other partner paraphrases the statement (**receiving partner/listener**).
- Confirmation from the sending partner is given that the communication was received accurately (paraphrase correct).
- The receiving partner becomes the sending partner.

For example:

WIFE: When we go for a walk together, I feel we are sharing something special.

HUSBAND: Our taking walks is a special time just for us.

WIFE: Yes.

HUSBAND: I don't enjoy walking as much as riding bikes together.

WIFE: You don't enjoy spending time with me.

HUSBAND: No. I enjoy spending time together, but I enjoy riding bikes together more.

WIFE: Oh. You like to ride bikes together versus walking together.

HUSBAND: That's right.

**Stress to the couple that:**

1. Understanding *does not* equal agreement. Paraphrasing what someone says does not mean that you agree with it, just that you heard and understood the message.
2. Paraphrasing can help you to identify what you *do* agree with and specify those areas of disagreement.
3. An incorrect paraphrase can be useful because it gives you an opportunity to restate yourself until your partner understands.
4. There is no single correct way to paraphrase; the important element is to communicate that you listened and understood.
5. It is often useful to shorten communication turns, and use more turns, to improve listening. This is often referred to as "speaking in paragraphs" (i.e., two to three bullet points that are easy for the listener to summarize) as opposed to "essays." This is especially true when discussing distressing topics or when one partner is prone to attention/concentration problems and/or dissociation. Taking in smaller chunks of shared information is more beneficial than taking in large chunks of unheard information.

### *In-Session Practice*

Have the couple turn their chairs to face each other to practice using the listening and paraphrasing skills. You will be using the skills to discuss content relevant to the psychoeducation on avoidance and intimate relationship functioning presented previously. Begin with the question:

*What has PTSD made us avoid? Talk about the people, places, things, or feelings that PTSD makes you avoid.*

The second question to be addressed using their listening/paraphrasing skills is:

*What would we do if we avoided less?*

These questions are designed to externalize the PTSD so that the couple can join around it to combat avoidance, diminish the likelihood of blaming behavior, and encourage approach behavior. We recommend that you have the PTSD+ partner begin the practice, with the other partner paraphrasing. Allow the couple to discuss the first topic for about 5 minutes, and the balance of the time available should be spent on envisioning a life without trauma-related avoidance.

While the couple is discussing, you should actively coach them in these paraphrasing skills. It is important to note that you **will likely need to be assertive in having each member of the couple paraphrase before making a statement**. When you prompt them to paraphrase what each other said (e.g., "Bob, what did you hear Mary say?"), the listening partner may respond to you instead of the speaking partner (e.g., "She said that we avoid going to the mall because crowds make her uncomfortable"). In this case, you can gently shape the couple to respond to each other instead of to you by saying, "I'll let you tell her what you heard her say."

You should also record on the *Avoidance List* (Handout 3.2) the people, places, things, and feelings that the couple discusses in order to help jump-start their completion of this assignment. *Figure 3.1* provides an example of Susan and Jake's avoidance list. As noted, because of Susan's anxiety, the couple avoided numerous places (e.g., bus stops, malls), situations (e.g., drinking beer socially, physical contact of any kind), people (e.g., men in general but especially those wearing baseball hats), and feelings (e.g., anger, fear). While recording these responses, the therapist noticed that all of these feared contexts were in some way reminiscent of Susan's trauma and provoked the same fight-or-flight response as during the rape. As a result, Susan avoided them, and to assuage her anxiety Jake "accommodated" Susan's PTSD symptoms by avoiding them too.

Be aware of the possibility of cognitive difficulties or more general methods of avoidance as you observe the couple's communication. Methods to overcome these challenges to communication include asking the couple to take shorter turns before paraphrasing, using each other's names more frequently (our focus in a conversation increases with the mention of our name), and prompting them to ask each other what the other heard them say if there are signs that the other may have "checked out." It is helpful for you to role-model how to ask the other cooperatively (vs. patronizingly) what he or she heard the partner say (e.g., "It seems like you might have left me for a second. Can you tell me what you heard?").

## Out-of-Session Assignments

Orient the couple to the *OOSA summary* (Handout 3.3) for this session and point out the following assignments:

- Continue to monitor positive behaviors in each other, even though they will not be asked to record these behaviors on a daily basis.
- Read over **together** *PTSD and Avoidance* (Handout 3.1) prior to the next session.

**List below as many things as possible that you, as a couple or individually, avoid but would approach if PTSD took up less space in your relationship.**

| Places | Situations |
|---|---|
| bus stops | drinking beer in the presence of others |
| malls | going out alone after dark |
| grocery stores | going out without pepper spray |
| parking lots | any physical contact, especially sex |

| People | Feelings |
|---|---|
| men wearing baseball hats | anger |
| but also men in general | fear |
| | sadness |
| | happiness |

**FIGURE 3.1.** Susan and Jake's Avoidance List.

- Together, continue identifying people, places, things, and feelings that the PTSD+ partner and the couple avoid. This *Avoidance List* (*Handout 3.2*) will be used throughout the rest of the therapy to develop *in vivo* approach assignments for the couple. See *Figure 3.1* as an example of a completed *Avoidance List*.
- On a daily basis, have each partner catch the other paraphrasing (*Handout 3.3*). The couple should record either the content of the paraphrase or the presence of paraphrasing each day. In other words, they are other-monitoring, not self-monitoring, paraphrasing behavior.

## Check-Out

Ask the couple how the session was for each of them. Are there any lingering concerns or questions? What do they want to take with them from the session? Infuse hopefulness and predict success in completing the OOSAs as they leave the session.

HANDOUT 3.1

# PTSD and Avoidance

As we discussed in the session, many people who have experienced trauma try to avoid thoughts and feelings associated with that event. Similarly, many people also avoid situations, places, and activities that remind them of the trauma or because they feel scary. People with PTSD can also become frightened of the thoughts, feelings, and physical sensations associated with emotions. This tendency has been described as a "fear of feeling." Although avoiding can make you feel more comfortable in the short run, it actually can make the problem worse in the long run because it prevents you from overcoming your fears.

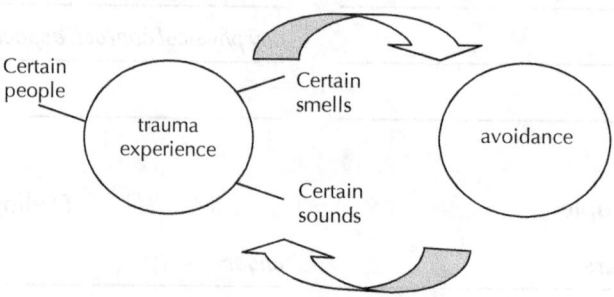

Like avoiding situations, places, and activities that remind them of traumas, people with PTSD come to avoid their own internal experiences, such as their thoughts, feelings, and physical sensations. We sometimes describe this as a fear of feeling. Techniques to avoid your inner experience might include being over-busy, thinking obsessively, numbing your emotions, overcontrolling your emotions for fear of being out of control, or injuring yourself to distract from painful emotions.

When you confront feared conversations, memories, situations, or feelings, several things begin to happen.

- Facing these situations **helps you make sense of them** (e.g., Why am I afraid to talk to my spouse about our children? → She might figure out that I don't feel like I'm an adequate parent).
- You learn that thinking about these experiences **is not dangerous and that being upset or anxious is not dangerous** (e.g., I won't go crazy if I'm sad after talking about these situations. In fact, my partner and I feel closer).
- You **become less fearful** of other situations that remind you of these situations (e.g., Now that I've faced this and had a positive experience, why wouldn't that be the case in the future?).
- You learn that you can **handle your fear and anxiety** and, therefore, you feel better about yourself (e.g., I'm strong enough to handle being sad or angry without acting on these feelings. I don't have to feel *good* all of the time, but rather be *good* at feeling).
- You learn that when you repeatedly confront memories or situations you have avoided, the fear and distress gradually decrease. In other words, you again become relatively comfortable in these situations (e.g., I don't get nearly as upset as I used to discussing these things with my partner).

Choosing to address more directly difficult issues for yourself and your relationship is hard work in the short term but will lead to long-term payoff.

---

From *Cognitive-Behavioral Conjoint Therapy for PTSD: Harnessing the Healing Power of Relationships* by Candice M. Monson and Steffany J. Fredman. Copyright 2012 by The Guilford Press. Permission to photocopy this handout is granted to purchasers of this book for personal use only (see copyright page for details).

HANDOUT 3.2

# Avoidance List

List below as many things as possible that you, as a couple or individually, avoid but would approach if PTSD took up less space in your relationship.

| Places | Situations |
| --- | --- |
| _____ | _____ |
| _____ | _____ |
| _____ | _____ |
| _____ | _____ |
| _____ | _____ |
| _____ | _____ |

| People | Feelings |
| --- | --- |
| _____ | _____ |
| _____ | _____ |
| _____ | _____ |
| _____ | _____ |
| _____ | _____ |
| _____ | _____ |

From *Cognitive-Behavioral Conjoint Therapy for PTSD: Harnessing the Healing Power of Relationships* by Candice M. Monson and Steffany J. Fredman. Copyright 2012 by The Guilford Press. Permission to photocopy this handout is granted to purchasers of this book for personal use only (see copyright page for details).

HANDOUT 3.3

# Out-of-Session Assignments
## Session 3. Listening and Approaching

1. Continue to watch for, and point out, **positive** behaviors in each other.
2. Read over the *PTSD and Avoidance* (Handout 3.1) together prior to your next session.
3. Together, continue to write down things on the *Avoidance List* (Handout 3.2) that we started in today's session that you seem to **avoid** in your day-to-day life. This list will be used in the rest of the therapy.
4. Each day prior to the next session, spend 5 minutes communicating with one another using your best paraphrasing skills. Each of you should notice if the other **paraphrased** in your communication. If so, place a checkmark in that person's column or write down the content of his or her paraphrasing. Put this form somewhere obvious for the two of you as a reminder to practice the skill in your day-to-day life.

**Next appointment:** _____ @ _____.

## CATCH EACH OTHER PARAPHRASING

Week of: _____

|  | Person Caught: _____ | Person Caught: _____ |
|---|---|---|
| **Example:** | concerns at work | ✓ |
| *Sunday* | | |
| *Monday* | | |
| *Tuesday* | | |
| *Wednesday* | | |
| *Thursday* | | |
| *Friday* | | |
| *Saturday* | | |

---

From *Cognitive-Behavioral Conjoint Therapy for PTSD: Harnessing the Healing Power of Relationships* by Candice M. Monson and Steffany J. Fredman. Copyright 2012 by The Guilford Press. Permission to photocopy this handout is granted to purchasers of this book for personal use only (see copyright page for details).

# SESSION 4

# Sharing Thoughts and Feelings
## Emphasis on *Feelings*

---

### SUMMARY OF SESSION CONTENT

#### Goals

- Teach the skill of channel checking.
- Improve the identification, experience, and expression of feelings in the dyadic context.

#### Key Interventions

1. Review of Out-of-Session Assignments
   - *Notice Positive Behaviors in Each Other*
   - *PTSD and Avoidance* (Handout 3.1)
   - *Avoidance List* (Handout 3.2)
   - *Catch Each Other Paraphrasing* (Handout 3.3)
2. Communication Channels (*Communication Channels*, Handout 4.1)
   - Introduce channel checking.
   - Illustrate the skill of channel checking.
3. Introduction to the Channel of Sharing Thoughts and Feelings (Focus on Feelings)
   - Provide rationale for sharing feelings.
   - Identifying feelings (*Identifying Feelings*, Handout 4.2).
   - Expressing feelings.
   - Reflecting feelings.
4. In-Session Practice of Sharing, with Emphasis on Feelings
   - The couple practices emotion expression skills to discuss how PTSD has affected them and their relationship.
   - Compare each partner's intimacy ratings from before and after the communication exercise.
5. Shrinking PTSD through Approach
   - Determine at least one person, place, situation, or feeling to be approached.
   - Maximizing effectiveness of approach tasks (*PROUD to Shrink PTSD*, Handout 4.3).
   - Record the item on the *OOSA summary* (Handout 4.4).
6. Out-of-Session Assignments (Handout 4.4)
   - *Notice Positive Behaviors in Each Other*
   - *Channel checking*
   - *PROUD to Shrink PTSD* (Handout 4.3)
   - *Catch Your Partner's Feelings* (Handout 4.4)
   - *Shrinking PTSD through Approach* (Handout 4.4)
7. Check-Out

*Administer the patient and partner versions of PCL/relationship happiness.

## Review of Out-of-Session Assignments

### *Positive Behaviors*

Inquire about positive behaviors that the couple has noticed in themselves and each other.

### *PTSD and Avoidance (Handout 3.1)*

Inquire whether either partner had any questions about this handout.

### *Avoidance List (Handout 3.2)*

Review the items that the couple added to the list of trauma-related places, people, things, and so on that they tend to avoid. Reinforce their hard work in identifying these areas and note that you will be using this list to help them shrink the role of PTSD in their lives throughout the rest of the therapy.

### *Catch Each Other Paraphrasing (Handout 3.3)*

Review the couple's success with catching each other paraphrasing in their out-of-session communication. Inquire whether there were instances in which the technique prevented misunderstanding. Inquire whether they enjoy having their partner "tuned into" what they are saying.

## Communication Channels

In this section, you will be helping the couple "get on the right channel" with each other. The following key points should be covered in this section while presenting *Communication Channels (Handout 4.1)*:

- Solicit personal examples from the couple in which they found themselves discussing something with their partner and thinking their partner did not seem to be responsive to what they were saying.

*Think of a time when you wanted to let your partner know how you felt about something. He or she, on the other hand, was telling you how you could solve or improve the situation.*

*You were in the **sharing** mode, while your partner was in the **solving** mode. You probably both got frustrated because you did not feel understood, and your partner might have felt rejected because you did not pursue his or her suggestions.*

- Verbal interactions have many purposes: to exchange information, pass the time of day, figure out your position, convey feelings, and so on.
- A primary task in any interaction is to identify the *goal* of the interaction, in other words to get on the same channel.

- There are two primary channels: *sharing thoughts and feelings* and *problem solving/decision making* (draw attention to the handout).
- The sharing channel usually "trumps" the solving channel. It is difficult for problem solving to occur until the person on the sharing channel feels heard. Sometimes it is necessary to switch to the problem-solving channel to address something in a timely manner (e.g., making decisions related to funeral arrangements). Nevertheless, the couple will likely need to return to the sharing channel following the necessitated switch to the problem-solving channel. Expect to switch back and forth at times; the important thing is working to be on the same channel during communication.

## *Illustrating the Skill of Channel Checking*

Channel checking can involve the receiving partner clarifying the goal of the communication when a message is sent.

*There are some very simple phrases that you might use to check the channel. For example, a wife says:*

> "What an awful day! I can't see how I can stand another day!"

*Her husband might say:*

> "Do you want me to listen or do you want some advice?"
> Or
> "Which channel are you on?"
> Or
> "It sounds like you just want to express your feelings about this right now."
> Or
> "It might be better for us to express our feelings about this before we try to come up with a solution."
> Or
> "Are we problem solving, or would you like to talk about what you're upset about?"

It is also important to instruct the couple that it is appropriate for the original sender of information to ask for what he or she wants in their communication when the partner does not seem to be on the same channel of communication.

*A wife might say:*

> "Right now I would just like to talk about what went on. I'm not ready to do anything about it."
> Or
> "I could use some help figuring out a solution to this problem."
> Or
> "Thanks for trying to help by offering solutions. I'm interested in just sharing for now."

# Introduction to the Channel of Sharing Thoughts and Feelings (Focus on Feelings)

Building on the skill of determining partners' communication channel, this session focuses on identifying, sharing, and reflecting feelings when the couple is on the sharing thoughts and feelings channel. PTSD can have corrosive effects on intimate relationships because of the PTSD-affected individual's fear of feeling and tendency to avoid emotions. Emotional numbing and distraction may be avoidant coping strategies that individuals with PTSD use to cope with their fear of feelings. As a result of emotional numbing, there may be individual difficulties in identifying and expressing both positive and negative emotions as well as relationship-level difficulties with intimacy. Shared emotional expression is one way that couples feel intimate and close to each other. To combat this fear of feeling, secondary emotional numbing, and the resulting difficulties with intimacy, the couple will have the opportunity to go through a set of dyadically oriented exercises designed to increase attention to the experience, expression, and reflection of feelings.

## *Identifying Feelings*

Research literature suggests that trauma survivors, in particular, can have difficulty with identifying, let alone expressing, their emotions to others (i.e., alexithymia; Price et al., 2006). Thus, *Identifying Feelings (Handout 4.2)* should be presented to the clients to help in expanding their repertoire of emotional language. Discuss the "primary colors" of feelings: mad, sad, scared, disgusted, ashamed, and glad (happy). These primary emotions are then blended to provide a variety of emotion "colors" and may be more or less intense in color.

> *There are some basic feelings that we know that people experience. Those emotions might be considered the "primary colors" of feelings. Like colors of the rainbow, these feelings can be mixed to develop other emotion colors. For example, a combination of mad and sad might yield disappointment. A combination of mad and scared might yield jealousy.*
>
> *There are various intensities to these colors too. For example, there is a continuum of mad:*
>
> *irritated → annoyed → angry → hostile → rageful*
>
> *And a continuum of scared:*
>
> *cautious → apprehensive → anxious → terrified*

## *Expressing Feelings*

The general principles about sharing feelings that should be discussed include:

1. The goal is not to get rid of negative emotions but rather to learn to tolerate, manage, and use them better.
2. Negative feelings can be as much of a "glue" in relationships as positive feelings. With exception of hostility, the expression of feelings seems to be what is most important.

3. There are no right or wrong feelings.
4. An easy opening statement for sharing of feelings is "I feel _____ [feeling word]."
5. To promote our loved ones telling us how they feel, it is important to provide a nonjudgmental environment for their expression.

### *Reflecting Feelings*

Reflection of feelings goes a step beyond paraphrasing to communicate to one's partner an understanding of his or her feelings. The reflection of feelings is important to truly *sharing* feelings. It is in the reflection that feelings become shared and empathy is fostered. An individual's reflections *mirror* the feelings the speaker seems to be expressing. Most people find it satisfying to have their partner reflect their emotions because this communicates understanding and support. It's nice to know that someone in the world is listening to us.

*Examples of reflection of feelings include:*

*"You sound really sad."*
*"That must have been exciting for you."*
*"You must be feeling frustrated by this."*
*"You're angry at Jim for his remarks to you."*

## In-Session Practice of Sharing, with Emphasis on Feelings

Prior to discussing the following two topics using reflection and emotion identification skills, ask each partner to **rate his or her sense of emotional intimacy with one another** on a 0–10 scale (0 = not close at all; 10 = as close as I can imagine) by inquiring, "How close do you feel to each other right now?" You can ask them to tell you verbally or write down their intimacy ratings individually and share the pre- and postintimacy ratings at the end of the communication practice. Demonstrating the **change** in intimacy as a result of sharing feelings is more important than the absolute intimacy experienced.

Ask the couple to turn their chairs to face each other and to use their reflecting and emotion identification skills to discuss the following two topics. As in last session, spend about 5 minutes on the first question before using the balance of the available time to pose the second question.

*What kinds of feelings does PTSD make you have?*

*When you imagine shrinking PTSD in your relationship, how does that make you feel?*

To facilitate couples using feeling words in the discussion, encourage them to refer to *Identifying Feelings (Handout 4.2)*. It is important to note that many patients with PTSD will have ambivalent feelings about shrinking the role of PTSD in their relationship (e.g., happy and scared). It is helpful to normalize this, especially for partners who will tend to have only positive emotions in response to imagining PTSD shrinking.

After these discussions, ask the couple to rate **their sense of emotional intimacy with one another** on the 0–10 scale. It is expected that intimacy will have increased as a result of the emotional communication. Point out that negative emotions arose in their discussion, yet their intimacy increased. Use this to reinforce the point that the process of sharing is more important than whether the emotion shared was positive or negative.

To enhance the probability of increasing intimacy, intervene swiftly at the onset of any hostile, critical, or blaming exchanges between the couple and join them together against PTSD versus one another. Slow the communication down with deliberate paraphrasing and elicit softer, more vulnerable emotions. If, in spite of these efforts, intimacy does not increase, first validate the couple for taking risks and then proceed to discuss what each was thinking and feeling during the conversation to figure out the point at which the communication took a negative turn. Use this as an opportunity to determine which skills would be helpful in future communication. Also, make sure to point out that this particular communication practice does not foretell the outcomes of future efforts, especially if they use their newly developing communication skills going forward.

## Shrinking PTSD through Approach

Remind the couple that an important element to shrinking the role of PTSD is approaching currently avoided people, places, and so on. The list of avoided people, places, situations, and things that the couple developed in and out of Session 3 will become the *Avoidance List (Handout 3.2)* to be used throughout the rest of the therapy. We developed *PROUD to Shrink PTSD (Handout 4.3)* to educate couples about the most essential ingredients of successful approach assignments in order to maximize their effectiveness. Review each of the concepts with the couple, making sure that they understand the principles.

- *Graduated and increasingly uncomfortable.* The exercises should be approached in a graduated manner such that each one pushes the couple out of their comfort zone but also provides a sense of mastery as they attempt increasingly difficult activities. Toward this end, guide the couple to pick a **moderately** distressing situation so that the therapy is efficiently delivered but maximizes the likelihood of success. In keeping with principles of exposure therapy for anxiety disorders outlined by Antony and Roemer (2011), we recommend that the approach activities be (1) predictable and under the couple's control but also (2) of sufficient duration and intensity so that the PTSD+ partner feels anxious or uncomfortable but then has the opportunity to experience what it feels like when the discomfort subsides. In most cases, couples should plan to devote 1–2 hours for each exercise, depending on the type of activity, and they should strive for activities that are challenging but doable.

We have not followed the convention of using SUDS (Subjective Units of Distress Scale) ratings to operationalize patients' distress before, during, and after approaching feared situations as is typical of exposure therapies for PTSD such as prolonged exposure (Foa et al., 2007). Instead, we have found that couples' learning to adopt a general strategy of approaching until their distress subsides rather than avoiding feared situations is sufficient to begin promoting a sense of safety and new learning. This strategy is also consistent with data suggesting that a certain decrease in SUDS within exposure sessions does not seem necessary to promote new learning across sessions (Baker et al., 2010).

- *Rewarding for the couple.* Approach activities that double as shared rewarding activities (e.g., going to movies, restaurants, social events, physical closeness) are often ideal because the couple is able to simultaneously shrink the presence of PTSD in their relationship and increase overall relationship satisfaction. For instance, one of us worked with a couple in which the PTSD+ partner, a Vietnam War veteran, avoided restaurants because he felt uncomfortable in crowded places. As a result, he and his wife were deprived of the opportunity to connect over nice dinners out and to socialize with others outside of their home. In this case, programming of the couple-level approach activities involved the couple going to restaurants at times when they were unlikely to be crowded (e.g., 2 P.M. on a Monday), and then going at times when they were likely to be increasingly busy (e.g., 5 P.M. on a Saturday and then 6 P.M., 7 P.M., and so on), all the while challenging themselves to sit closer to the center of the restaurant rather than toward the walls and having the PTSD+ partner sit with his back toward the inside of the restaurant instead of against the wall.

- *Variable stimuli to promote generalization.* To maximize gains, it is helpful to **vary stimuli** that provoke distress, applying approach behaviors **across multiple contexts**. For example, a rape survivor who was assaulted while at a college fraternity party feels anxious whenever she hears music from the 1980s, smells beer, or attends any kind of social gathering. In this case, the couple might be encouraged to listen to 1980s music on their way to a restaurant, where they will meet up with friends for happy hour and have a beer. To encourage generalization to feared situations, the next activity could involve playing 1980s music at their home while they host family and friends for a barbecue that involves serving beer in addition to other drinks and food.

- *Participate fully and without distraction.* For activities to be maximally beneficial, it is important that patients not "white knuckle" their way through them, because then no new learning has taken place; in this case, they have merely reinforced the idea that the only way to get through an uncomfortable situation is to brace themselves for the worst. Similarly, it is also key that couples fully participate in the activity and do not engage in distraction through the myriad behaviors that could take attention away from the activity itself (e.g., drinking, reading a magazine, talking on a cell phone). In fact, there may be cases in which partners and children serve as "safety signals" to help manage patients' anxiety through distraction or reassurance. To address this, it may be necessary to **think dyadically but intervene individually** by having loved ones initially involved in the approach activities but then gradually withdrawn as the patients move increasingly out of their comfort zones (see the case of Donna presented shortly).

Following are examples of couple-level approach activities structured in a graduated manner.

***Case example 1: Mark, an Iraq War combat veteran who avoided nearly all physical contact with his wife because of both emotional numbing and fears of intimacy***

| Step | Activity |
|---|---|
| 1 | *Hug daily* |
| 2 | *Kiss on cheek daily* |
| 3 | *Sit on couch next to each other daily* |
| 4 | *Hold hands daily while on couch* |

| 5 | Cuddle on couch daily |
| 6 | Go to bed at the same time daily |
| 7 | Massage daily |
| 8 | Kissing daily |
| 9 | Nongenital sexual touching daily |
| 10 | Sexual touching with no intercourse daily |

**Case example 2:** Donna, a motor vehicle accident survivor whose sister drove her wherever she needed to go because she felt anxious at the prospect of driving

| Step | Activity |
| --- | --- |
| 1 | Drive on own street with sister in passenger seat |
| 2 | Drive on own street with sister in back seat |
| 3 | Drive down several streets in neighborhood with sister in passenger seat |
| 4 | Drive down several streets in neighborhood with sister in back seat |
| 5 | Drive down several streets in neighborhood alone |
| 6 | Drive within neighborhood with sister in back seat |
| 7 | Drive within neighborhood alone |
| 8 | Drive to grocery store and back home with sister in back seat |
| 9 | Drive to grocery store and back home alone |
| 10 | Drive on highway with sister in passenger seat |
| 11 | Drive on highway with sister in back seat |
| 12 | Drive on highway alone |

To maximize gains during the relatively brief course of this treatment, encourage the couple to proceed through multiple steps of the approach hierarchy in between sessions. That is, once the couple has achieved success with an earlier step(s), they should challenge themselves to keep working on increasingly difficult tasks until those are also mastered. Thus, in the case of Mark just described, the couple might be able to complete Steps 1–4 (hugging to holding hands) in the span of 4–5 days or a week depending on how quickly they achieve comfort with each of the various intimate behaviors.

It is important for the couple to have success with this first assignment of *in vivo* approach behavior. Therefore, try to help them select an activity/situation that is challenging but reasonable to accomplish prior to the next session and, to the extent possible, anticipate, with the couple, barriers to the success of carrying out the approach behavior. For example, inform the couple that you anticipate that the PTSD+ partner is not going to want to do the task—and that this reluctance is the PTSD "talking." If it was easy, they would already be doing it. Ask questions such as, "What will you do at the moment that Betty does not want to approach the place that you've agreed to approach in this session? Are there things that we can think of now that we should put in place to help her approach despite feeling anxious in the moment?"

Session 4. Sharing Thoughts and *Feelings*

From the *Avoidance List* (*Handout 3.2*), determine at least one place, situation, or thing (not necessarily feelings, because of the daily feeling "catch") that will be approached prior to the next session. Record the item on the *OOSA summary* (*Handout 4.4*) and ask the couple to write a brief sentence or two describing how it went.

Anticipate with the couple barriers to the success of carrying out the approach behavior and preemptively problem solve how those behaviors might be overcome. Refer them to the PROUD acronym in *Handout 4.3* to help strategize maximizing the benefits of the approach exercise.

## Out-of-Session Assignments

Orient the couple to the *OOSA summary sheet* (*Handout 4.4*) for this session and point out the following assignments:

- Continue to monitor positive behaviors in each other, even though they will not be asked record these behaviors on a daily basis.
- Each member should practice a channel check at least once prior to the next session.
- Together, read over *PROUD to Shrink PTSD* (*Handout 4.3*).
- On a daily basis, have each partner catch the other expressing a feeling and record the feeling "caught" on the *OOSA summary sheet* (*Handout 4.4*).
- Complete at least one *in vivo* approach behavior off of the *Avoidance List* (*Handout 3.2*) to shrink PTSD.

## Check-Out

Ask the couple how the session was for each of them. Are there any lingering concerns or questions? What do they want to take with them from the session? Infuse hopefulness and predict success in completing the OOSAs as they leave the session.

## HANDOUT 4.1
# Communication Channels

### CHANNEL CHECK

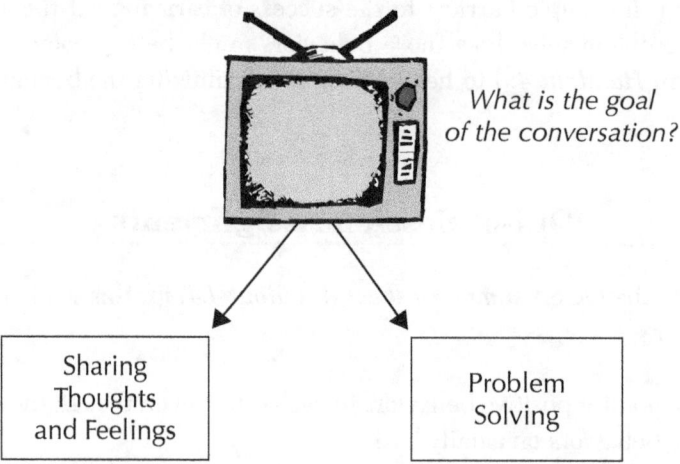

The first step in effective communication is to check your channels. Knowing about the different channels of communication can help you determine the *goal* of the conversation. What channel are you on? Do you want to solve a problem, or do you want to share about it? What channel is your partner on? Are you on the same channel? As partners, you will have greater understanding of one another and more satisfaction in your communication if you become aware of what the difference is between the channels and notice the channels each of you are on. For instance, one partner may be on the sharing channel and wants to be understood rather than to work out the details of problem solving. Or one partner is on the problem-solving channel and is eager to resolve a particular issue. When couples are on different channels—that is, when one person is on the solving channel and the other is on the sharing channel—conflict, confusion, and miscommunication can result. Checking in to see which channels you are on can open the door to understanding, intimacy, empathy, and improved conflict resolution.

---

From *Cognitive-Behavioral Conjoint Therapy for PTSD: Harnessing the Healing Power of Relationships* by Candice M. Monson and Steffany J. Fredman. Copyright 2012 by The Guilford Press. Permission to photocopy this handout is granted to purchasers of this book for personal use only (see copyright page for details).

# HANDOUT 4.2
# Identifying Feelings

|  | Feelings (intensity) | Thought |
|---|---|---|
|  | 0　　　　　　　　50　　　　　　　　100 |  |
| Mad | *irritated* → annoyed → angry → hostile → rageful | Unfairness |
| Sad | *down* → glum → depressed → miserable → despondent | Loss |
| Scared | *cautious* → apprehensive → anxious → terrified | Danger |
| Disgusted | *a little turned off* → appalled → revolted | Contamination/violation |
| Ashamed | *embarrassed* → disgraced → humiliated → mortified | Self as bad |
| Glad | *contented* → pleased → happy → delighted → ecstatic | Self, others, or world as positive |
| Horrified | scared + disgusted | Danger + Contamination |
| Jealous | mad + scared | Unfairness + Danger |
| Disappointed | mad + sad | Unfairness + Loss |

From *Cognitive-Behavioral Conjoint Therapy for PTSD: Harnessing the Healing Power of Relationships* by Candice M. Monson and Steffany J. Fredman. Copyright 2012 by The Guilford Press. Permission to photocopy this handout is granted to purchasers of this book for personal use only (see copyright page for details).

HANDOUT 4.3

# PROUD to Shrink PTSD
## Getting the Most Out of Your Approach Tasks

### P = PLANNED

*Approach tasks should be **planned**.* Decide in advance what you will approach. Plan together in advance when you will complete your practice assignment and put it in your schedule. Have a backup plan in case the original plan doesn't work out.

### R = REPEAT, REPEAT, REPEAT

*Successful approach tasks are **repeated** frequently.* The more you approach what you have avoided, the more you will learn. It is a good idea to practice being in the same situation *repeatedly* until it becomes easier.

### O = OBSTACLES

*Remove **obstacles** to your new learning.* Sometimes people will put themselves in approach situations, but find ways to avoid during them and, therefore, not learn. You may distract yourself, drink alcohol or use drugs, rely on your partner or children to help you through the situation, or "white knuckle" through the experience (i.e., just getting through the situation without really being there). Try to avoid doing anything that might prevent your new learning!

### U = UNCOMFORTABLE

*Expect to feel **uncomfortable**.* It is perfectly normal to feel distressed while you are doing approach assignments. This is why they are on the approach list! Success should not be judged by how you felt in the situation. Rather, success should be judged by whether you were able to feel your feelings and stay in the situation.

### D = DECREASE DISTRESS

*Stay in the situation until your distress decreases.* In order for you to learn new information from your experiences, it is very important for you to stay in the situation long enough to learn from it. Your distress is not likely to completely subside, but stay in the situation as long as you can to notice it decrease.

---

From *Cognitive-Behavioral Conjoint Therapy for PTSD: Harnessing the Healing Power of Relationships* by Candice M. Monson and Steffany J. Fredman. Copyright 2012 by The Guilford Press. Permission to photocopy this handout is granted to purchasers of this book for personal use only (see copyright page for details).

HANDOUT 4.4

# Out-of-Session Assignments

## Session 4. Sharing Thoughts and Feelings: Emphasis on Feelings

1. Continue to watch for, and point out, positive behaviors in each other.
2. **Each of you** practices a channel check at least once prior to the next session.
3. At least one time per day, catch your partner sharing a feeling. Record the feeling "caught" below. You may need to ask how he or she is feeling in order to catch a feeling.
4. Shrinking PTSD through Approach: _____

   (people, place, situation, feeling)

   Write about how it went:
   _____
   _____

   Place this form somewhere that is convenient and visible to the two of you.

**Next appointment:** _____ @ _____.

### CATCH YOUR PARTNER'S FEELINGS

Week of: _____

| | *Partner* _____ | *Partner* _____ |
|---|---|---|
| **Example:** *Tuesday* | *annoyed* | *happy* |
| Sunday | | |
| Monday | | |
| Tuesday | | |
| Wednesday | | |
| Thursday | | |
| Friday | | |
| Saturday | | |

---

From *Cognitive-Behavioral Conjoint Therapy for PTSD: Harnessing the Healing Power of Relationships* by Candice M. Monson and Steffany J. Fredman. Copyright 2012 by The Guilford Press. Permission to photocopy this handout is granted to purchasers of this book for personal use only (see copyright page for details).

# SESSION 5

# Sharing Thoughts and Feelings
## Emphasis on *Thoughts*

---

**SUMMARY OF SESSION CONTENT**

### Goals

- Introduce the role of thoughts in emotions and behaviors.
- Plant the seed that thoughts are malleable and can be changed to improve PTSD and relationship satisfaction.
- Set the stage for effective dyadic cognitive intervention in the final phases of therapy focused on the trauma(s) appraisals.

### Key Interventions

1. Review of Out-of-Session Assignments
   - Notice Positive Behaviors in Each Other
   - Channel Checking
   - PROUD to Shrink PTSD (*Handout 4.3*)
   - Catch Your Partner's Feelings (*Handout 4.4*)
   - Shrinking PTSD through Approach (*Handout 4.4*)
2. Identifying Thoughts on the Sharing Channel (*Sharing Thoughts and Feelings to Shrink PTSD, Handout 5.1*)
   - Increase awareness of thoughts and their expression.
   - Explain the associations among thoughts, feelings, and behaviors.
3. In-Session Practice
   - The couple practices expressing thoughts and related feelings regarding how PTSD has affected them and their relationship.
   - Compare each partner's intimacy ratings from before and after the communication exercise.
4. Shrinking PTSD through Approach
   - Determine at least one person, place, situation, or feeling to be approached.
   - Record the item on the *OOSA summary* (*Handout 5.3*).
5. Out-of-Session Assignments (*Handout 5.3*)
   - Notice Positive Behaviors in Each Other
   - Sharing Thoughts and Feelings to Shrink PTSD (*Handout 5.1*)
   - Catch Your Partner's Thoughts and Feelings (*Handout 5.2*)
   - Shrinking PTSD through Approach (*Handout 5.3*)
6. Check-Out

*Administer the patient and partner versions of PCL/relationship happiness.

## Review of Out-of-Session Assignments

### *Positive Behaviors*

Inquire about positive behaviors that the couple has noticed in themselves and their partner.

### *Channel Checking*

Inquire whether both members of the couple did a channel check in their communication. If so, how was it helpful? If not, what got in the way?

### *PROUD to Shrink PTSD (Handout 4.3)*

Inquire whether either of the partners had any questions about this handout.

### *Catch Your Partner's Feelings (Handout 4.4)*

In reviewing the responses to this *OOSA*, consider the following:

1. Was there was a range of emotions, both negative and positive, expressed within the couple's relationship? If so, highlight this to the couple and reinforce them for being so attuned to each other in this manner. If not, comment on whether there tended to be a particular emotion that was more frequently expressed (e.g., anger) and inquire what it would be like to express and notice other emotions (e.g., sadness, happiness, fear). Predict for them that, with practice, they will start to experience and notice many different kinds of feelings and that this will help them to feel closer to one another.
2. Was there a tendency to express certain types of emotions over others (e.g., anger vs. more vulnerable emotions)? If so, ask them to experiment with expressing an emotion that they do not usually express or that makes them feel slightly uncomfortable in the spirit of approaching rather than avoiding.
3. How rich and precise are the words that they used to describe their emotions expressed? In particular, the more nuanced the words used (e.g., *annoyed* to indicate a mild level of anger vs. *upset*), the more emotional numbing will be decreased and emotional intimacy increased.
4. What was the effect of sharing more emotions in their relationship? Again, highlight the notion that sharing emotions increases emotional intimacy, even if negative emotions were shared.

Your goal is to expand the valence, range, and repertoire of emotion words that the couple uses in their relationship. If you notice any improvement that could be made in those different aspects of emotion expression, encourage the couple to continue work on this area, in conjunction with the current session's OOSA (*Handout 5.3*), which includes monitoring of the association between thoughts and feelings.

### Shrinking PTSD through Approach (Handout 4.4)

Review how the *in vivo* assignment went and reinforce any approach behavior and couple-level facilitation of such. Troubleshoot ways in which the couple may have accommodated avoidance. If the couple was successful in approaching an item off of the *Avoidance List (Handout 3.2)*, in some way note this on their list (e.g., cross it out if no longer avoided, place a checkmark if previously assigned but still working on it).

## Identifying Thoughts on the Sharing Channel

To help reinforce the different types of communication that the couple may have, remind them that this session is still related to the channel regarding *sharing versus solving*. It may be helpful to orient them to *Communication Channels (Handout 4.1)* from their binder, highlighting the two types of communication. This session focuses on sharing thoughts as well as their relationship to feelings. Point out that this session builds upon the prior session by focusing on the thoughts that precede feeling states.

Many people are not aware of the ongoing thoughts that they have throughout their daily waking life, let alone share those thoughts with their intimate partners. Your goal is to increase awareness of thoughts and encourage the expression of them. Use the graphic in *Sharing Thoughts and Feelings to Shrink PTSD (Handout 5.1)* to illustrate the relationship between thoughts and feelings.

*Thus far in the therapy we have been working on your behavior and emotions. All of us have ongoing commentary in our minds about events, people, and places that we encounter, even if we aren't aware of those thoughts. It is one way that we are essentially human.*

*Sharing our thoughts about ourselves, others, and things that are happening in the world help us to know other people better. It lets us into another person's "head" to know more about them. In order to share one's thoughts, we have to become more aware of the thoughts that one is even having.*

*What we feel and how we act are highly dependent on what we are thinking. I'm sure you've been in a situation in which two or more people experienced the exact same thing and yet had very different interpretations of it. [Solicit example from the couple if possible, or use the example of different feelings that might result from different interpretations about the therapist not coming to get the couple from the waiting room (e.g., "He stood us up?" vs. "Maybe there was an emergency?" vs. "Did we get the appointment time wrong?").] This points to the power of perception, or how we think about situations, others, and ourselves in influencing our feelings.*

*Even though we are usually first aware of our feelings and actions, thoughts about a situation, ourselves, or our loved ones actually come before feelings and actions. These feelings and actions have positive and/or negative consequences for ourselves and our relationships. In this way, thoughts lead to feelings and actions.*

*event → thoughts → emotions → behaviors → consequences (+/−)*

## Session 5. Sharing *Thoughts* and Feelings

In a healthy relationship, one thing a partner does for us is to help **figure out** our thoughts. Sharing thoughts also helps them to understand us better and helps us to understand ourselves better. By sharing, rather than mind reading, we are in a better position to know each other better. *Catch Your Partner's Thoughts and Feelings* (Handout 5.2) will be assigned as an OOSA to help the couple avoid mind reading and to become more aware of their own and their partner's thoughts and related feelings.

Point out how PTSD can contribute to people thinking that they're under **threat**. Solicit examples from the couple about how threat-related cognitions as a result of PTSD have played out in their relationship. Highlight that these threat-related cognitions are more likely to contribute to relationship distress when the partner is not aware of what the traumatized person is thinking (e.g., Peter does not want to go to the movies because he is afraid that someone could set off a bomb in a crowded place, but Jane interprets his not wanting to go as a reflection of his not wanting to spend time with her). Thus, one of the goals of this session is to help partners become aware of each other's thoughts and associated feelings.

### In-Session Practice

Like last session, prior to discussing the following two topics using their developing communication skills, ask the partners to rate their sense of emotional intimacy with one another on a 0–10 scale (0 = not close at all; 10 = as close as I can imagine) by inquiring, "How close do you feel to each other right now?"

Ask the couple to turn their chairs to face each other and to use their communication skills to discuss the following two topics. Similar to the previous sessions, spend about 5 minutes on the first question before using the balance of the available time to pose the second question.

> *What kinds of thoughts and related feelings does PTSD make you have?*
>
> *When you imagine shrinking PTSD in your relationship, what specific thoughts and related feelings do you have?*

Examples of the kinds of thoughts that you hope to elicit include:

1. My family and I are unsafe. (PTSD-+ partner)
2. I can't handle crowds. (PTSD-+ partner)
3. I have to be in control. (PTSD-+ partner)
4. I have to walk on eggshells, or I'll provoke him. (partner)
5. I can't trust his emotions. (partner)
6. We can't be close. (partner)

Postpractice, ask the couple to rate their sense of emotional intimacy with one another on the 0–10 scale. Done well, intimacy will have increased as a result of the thoughts and feelings communication, even if negative emotions were shared.

Use the suggestions offered in the last session to promote success with the communication practice and to troubleshoot if intimacy does not increase.

## Shrinking PTSD through Approach

From the *Avoidance List* (Handout 3.2), determine the next place, situation, thing, or feeling that will be approached prior to the next session. It may be that the next approach behaviors will build on prior approach behaviors to successively approximate the fully desired approach behavior (e.g., Session 4: go to a restaurant during a busy time but sit in the corner or during a slow time and sit toward the middle; Session 5: go during a busy time and sit in the middle of the restaurant).

Record the item on the *OOSA summary* (Handout 5.3), and ask the couple to write about how it went.

As in the last session, anticipate with the couple barriers to the success of carrying out the approach behavior and preemptively problem solve how those behaviors might be overcome. Refer them to the PROUD acronym in *Handout 4.3* to help strategize maximizing the benefits of the approach exercise.

## Out-of-Session Assignments

Orient the couple to the *OOSA summary* (Handout 5.3) for this session and point out the following assignments:

- Continue to monitor positive behaviors in each other, even though they will not be asked to record these behaviors on a daily basis.
- Read together *Sharing Thoughts and Feelings to Shrink PTSD* (Handout 5.1).
- Allow time in this session to explain sufficiently the use of *Catch Your Partner's Thoughts and Feelings* (Handout 5.2). If possible, use a thought and feeling that emerged during the in-session communication practice and record it on the form so the couple can gain direct experience in its use.
- Remind the couple of the item chosen from the *Avoidance List* (Handout 3.2) to be approached prior to the next session and ask them to record how it went.

## Check-Out

Ask the couple how the session was for each of them. Are there any lingering concerns or questions? What do they want to take with them from the session to improve their relationship and PTSD? Infuse hopefulness and predict success in completing the OOSAs as they leave the session.

## HANDOUT 5.1
# Sharing Thoughts and Feelings to Shrink PTSD

As we discussed in today's session, what we feel and how we act are highly dependent on what we think. **Our perceptions** are very important. This is true for everyone, whether traumatized or not. You have probably had the experience of being in the same situation with other people only to find that they have a completely different story about the situation than you do. This happens because each person *perceives* differently. People organize what they see and hear into their own understanding of the situation.

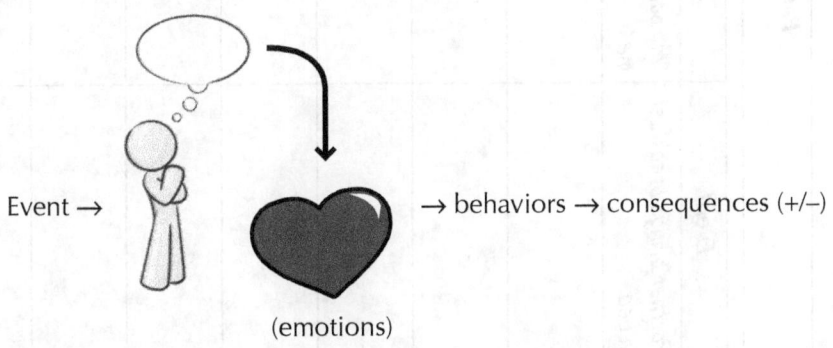

Event → → behaviors → consequences (+/–)

(emotions)

When an event occurs, there are thoughts or interpretations about that event. The way that you perceive or think about a situation influences feelings and behaviors. In this way, thoughts *lead* to feelings and actions. Sometimes, though, our thoughts are so **automatic** that we don't even realize that a thought came before our feeling or our action. Even though you may not be aware of what you are thinking or saying to yourself, your thoughts and self-talk affect your mood and your behavior. The goal of this therapy is to begin to recognize those automatic thoughts, to share them with your partner, and to notice how they make you feel and act.

Let's take an example. If someone with PTSD does not want to go somewhere (e.g., the movies) because he has the thought, "It's an open, dangerous place," he would likely have the feeling of fear and the urge to avoid. If he does not share this thought with his partner, the partner might have the thought, "We don't go places together because he doesn't care about me or want to spend time together," and feel hurt and angry. The partner may initiate an argument or withdraw. If the couple is able to talk about the thoughts and feelings that they are each having, there is greater understanding (and decreased miscommunication) and greater opportunity to consider shrinking PTSD by approaching the event rather than avoiding. An added benefit is that they will also feel closer as a couple.

---

From *Cognitive-Behavioral Conjoint Therapy for PTSD: Harnessing the Healing Power of Relationships* by Candice M. Monson and Steffany J. Fredman. Copyright 2012 by The Guilford Press. Permission to photocopy this handout is granted to purchasers of this book for personal use only (see copyright page for details).

HANDOUT 5.2

# Catch Your Partner's Thoughts and Feelings

Week of: _____

| | Partner: _____ | | | Partner: _____ | | |
|---|---|---|---|---|---|---|
| | Event | Thought | Feeling | Event | Thought | Feeling |
| Example: | Hear a noise outside | "Someone is trying to break in." | Afraid | Partner brings breakfast in bed. | "My partner cares about me." | Content |
| Sunday | | | | | | |
| Monday | | | | | | |
| Tuesday | | | | | | |
| Wednesday | | | | | | |
| Thursday | | | | | | |
| Friday | | | | | | |
| Saturday | | | | | | |

From *Cognitive-Behavioral Conjoint Therapy for PTSD: Harnessing the Healing Power of Relationships* by Candice M. Monson and Steffany J. Fredman. Copyright 2012 by The Guilford Press. Permission to photocopy this handout is granted to purchasers of this book for personal use only (see copyright page for details).

HANDOUT 5.3

# Out-of-Session Assignments

## Session 5. Sharing Thoughts and Feelings: Emphasis on Thoughts

1. Continue to watch for, and point out, positive behaviors in each other.
2. Read together *Sharing Thoughts and Feelings to Shrink PTSD* (Handout 5.1).
3. At least one time per day, catch a thought and feeling that your partner has in reaction to a situation. Record these on the *Catch Your Partner's Thoughts and Feelings* (Handout 5.2). At least one of the thoughts should be PTSD related. Notice the effects of sharing your thoughts and feelings with each other.
4. Shrinking PTSD through Approach:

_____

(people, place, situation, feeling)

Write about how it went:

_____
_____

Place this form somewhere that is convenient and visible to the two of you.

**Next appointment:** _____ @ _____

---

From *Cognitive-Behavioral Conjoint Therapy for PTSD: Harnessing the Healing Power of Relationships* by Candice M. Monson and Steffany J. Fredman. Copyright 2012 by The Guilford Press. Permission to photocopy this handout is granted to purchasers of this book for personal use only (see copyright page for details).

# SESSION 6

# Getting U.N.S.T.U.C.K.

---

**SUMMARY OF SESSION CONTENT**

### Goals

- Introduce and practice dyadic cognitive intervention with the U.N.S.T.U.C.K. process.

### Key Interventions

1. Review of Out-of-Session Assignments
   - *Notice Positive Behaviors in Each Other*
   - *Sharing Thoughts and Feelings to Shrink PTSD* (Handout 5.1)
   - *Catch Your Partner's Thoughts and Feelings* (Handout 5.2)
   - *Shrinking PTSD through Approach* (Handout 5.3)
2. Introduction to the U.N.S.T.U.C.K. Process (*Getting U.N.S.T.U.C.K.*, Handout 6.1)
   - Provide rationale for using the U.N.S.T.U.C.K. process.
   - Explain the steps of the U.N.S.T.U.C.K. process.
   - Introduce *The Big Picture* (Handout 6.2) to facilitate the U.N.S.T.U.C.K. process.
3. In-Session Practice of the U.N.S.T.U.C.K. Process
   - Guide the couple through at least one U.N.S.T.U.C.K. process using a thought held by the PTSD+ patient.
   - If time permits, do an additional U.N.S.T.U.C.K. process using a thought held by the partner.
4. Shrinking PTSD through Approach
   - Determine at least one person, place, situation, or feeling to be approached.
   - Record the item on the *OOSA summary* (Handout 6.4).
5. Out-of-Session Assignments (Handout 6.4)
   - *Notice Positive Behaviors in Each Other*
   - *The Big Picture* (Handout 6.2)
   - *Catch Your Partner's Thoughts and Feelings* (Handout 6.3)
   - *Shrinking PTSD through Approach* (Handout 6.4)
6. Check-Out

---

**\*Administer the patient and partner versions of PCL/relationship happiness.**

## Review of Out-of-Session Assignments

- *Positive Behaviors.* Inquire about positive behaviors that both members of the couple have noticed in themselves and in their partner.
- *Sharing Thoughts and Feelings to Shrink PTSD (Handout 5.1).* Inquire whether either partner had any questions about this handout.
- *Catch Your Partner's Thoughts and Feelings (Handout 5.2).* In reviewing the responses to this OOSA, consider the following:

1. Are thoughts identified as thoughts and feelings identified as feelings (i.e., are they reported in the correct column)? If not, use a recent event that occurred since the last session to coach the couple through this distinction.
2. Is there a tendency for a theme of thoughts and feelings?
3. Were both a trauma-related thought and a trauma-related feeling recorded? What was the nature of the thought and the feeling? How was it for the couple to approach trauma-related cognitions and feelings more explicitly?
4. What was it like for the couple to share thoughts with their partner? Were they surprised to learn what their partner was thinking about a certain event or topic, especially if it was different from their own thoughts?
5. What kinds of emotions did they observe in response to their thoughts?

Your goal is to highlight two points: **(1) Thoughts influence emotions and different thoughts can lead to different emotions; and (2) partners' thoughts can differ even though they've experienced the same event.**

- *Shrinking PTSD through Approach (Handout 5.3).* Review how the *in vivo* assignment went and reinforce any approach behavior and couple-level facilitation of such. Troubleshoot ways in which the couple may have accommodated avoidance. If the couple was successful in approaching an item off of the *Avoidance List* (Handout 3.2), in some way note this on their list (e.g., cross it out if no longer avoided, place a checkmark if previously assigned but still working on it).

## Introduction to the U.N.S.T.U.C.K. Process

We developed a new method of conducting cognitive interventions within the conjoint frame, called the U.N.S.T.U.C.K. process (see *Getting U.N.S.T.U.C.K.* [Handout 6.1]). The purpose of the U.N.S.T.U.C.K. process is to provide a set of steps that the couple can use together to challenge the ways in which they make sense of day-to-day events and later in appraising traumatic events and reactions to symptoms.

Contrary to traditional cognitive restructuring techniques (e.g., Beck, 1976), we developed this process to take into account advances from neuroscience and learning research (Bouton, 2000, 2004; Craske et al., 2008). More specifically, we built a process that emphasizes *cognitive flexibility* over thought modification, because it does not seem that thoughts are restructured per se. Rather, old learning (i.e., maladaptive thoughts) seems to exist in the presence of new learning (i.e., alternative, more functional thoughts). In this way, it may be better to think of the goal of cognitive interventions as being to "dilute" maladaptive attributions or appraisals rather than to change them. It also helps decrease any resistance that comes with people feeling forced to give up their original thoughts.

We also questioned the need for clients to learn **different types of thinking errors** in order to get to the ultimate goal of alternative perspectives. It has been our experience that clients, especially those of lower intelligence, literacy, or education, can be intimated by the logic focus and the similarity to academic work. They can also get tangled up in trying to identify the type of distortion, which may not be important to developing an alternative. This is not to say that clinicians do not benefit from knowing these characteristic thinking problems in order to guide the couple toward healthier thinking. However, our experience with the method and our research data indicate that couples do not need to know different types of thinking errors in order to benefit from the intervention.

In developing the intervention, we also sought to **decrease reliance on worksheets**. We wanted to create a process that could be *facilitated* by, but not reliant on, a particular form. Necessary paperwork might or might not be available when needed. Because of this, *The Big Picture* (*Handout 6.2*) is purposefully simple in its graphic design for re-creation on a blank piece of paper whenever and wherever desired. It was also designed to facilitate learning by including visual and verbal media. Thus, we incorporated "big picture" and "panoramic" thinking and the notion of writing alternative thoughts outside of the center "bubble." These notions are described shortly.

A final note about the U.N.S.T.U.C.K. process is that, contrary to more traditional methods of cognitive restructuring, we do not presume that a cognitive "error" or "distortion" will be noticed or needs to be noticed. The U.N.S.T.U.C.K. process is designed to facilitate critical thinking and evaluation of ways of thinking. In this vein, stress to the couple that sometimes thoughts are *not* a product of tunnel vision but are, in fact, based on good evidence. Nevertheless, the U.N.S.T.U.C.K. process can be used, and testing will reveal that the thought is relatively balanced, functional, and accurate. Problem-solving/decision-making skills to be taught in the next session can then ensue based on the realistic appraisals or attributions.

The steps of the U.N.S.T.U.C.K. process convey the major principles to be conveyed (see the following discussion).

Explain the steps of the U.N.S.T.U.C.K. process with the couple by showing them *Getting U.N.S.T.U.C.K.* (*Handout 6.1*). In introducing the dyadic cognitive intervention process, it is very important to engender a spirit of **collaboration, nonjudgmentalness, and open-mindedness**. The idea is to join the couple together in **collaborative empiricism** (Tee & Kazantzis, 2011).

Remind the couple that one of the most important roles that a partner fulfills in a healthy, happy relationship is one of reality testing. Partners help us determine whether our ways of thinking are eschewed and/or helpful.

## U.N.S.T.U.C.K. *Procedure*

*In prior sessions we have discussed how different people can have different thoughts about the same situation. We've also seen that different thoughts lead to different emotions. In today's session, we are going to take the power of our thoughts to the next level.*

*A very important role that partners serve in healthy relationships is to help one another evaluate whether the way that they are seeing things is accurate or helpful. In this way, healthy couples share their thoughts and feelings and join together like a scientific team to evaluate the evidence for their "truths."*

*Today I am going to teach you a process that you can use as a couple to be that collaborative team for each other. The first step to always remember is that you are on the same team—that is the U. You are **united** as a team. Our thoughts are very personal to us, and this process of evaluating them can thus feel very personal. It is important to remember that your **thoughts do not define you; you define your thoughts**. And you can always choose to change your mind.*

*The next step is to **notice and share** your thoughts. It is very helpful to boil down your thoughts to one or two primary thoughts about the issue. A helpful self-summary or paraphrase is, "So the bottom line is that you think _____."*

*The next step is to **brainstorm** the range of different thoughts that you might have about the situation. This is really a time to think "outside of box"—or outside of the bubble as it were. This is the time to try and see the biggest vision possible. It is okay if you don't necessarily believe everything you write down. The key is to open your minds. Both of you nominate or offer thoughts to be written down.*

*The next step is where you **test** the thoughts that you brainstormed. With a range of thoughts to be considered, what is the evidence for them? Is one or more of them more helpful?*

*The next step is to **use** the most balanced of them. Which of them are the most balanced and realistic?*

*The final two steps are particularly important. With a possible change of mind, how does that **change** your emotions and behavior? It is important to envision the effect of different thoughts on your feelings and actions.*

*Finally, you have likely been thinking certain ways for a long time. You have some well-worn paths of thinking, and like blazing a new path, changing your thoughts is going to take some work. At first, it is not going to be automatic at all. It will be very effortful, but with that effort, you will get the payoff. Thus, you're likely going to need to keep practicing. How would you test those new thoughts out with practice? How will you keep practicing those balanced thoughts?*

After describing each of the steps, present the couple with *The Big Picture* (Handout 6.2). This worksheet is designed to facilitate the U.N.S.T.U.C.K. process. It is a visual method to help the couple brainstorm the range of thoughts that might be had about a situation. *The Big Picture* begins with the step of noticing thoughts. The primary thought that is noticed and shared is written in the center (tunnel) of the page. The couple is instructed that there is a tendency for all of us to have "tunnel vision" at times, not necessarily seeing the big picture.

Alternative thoughts are nominated by both members of the couple and are written outside of the tunnel (S) and subsequently tested for evidence and healthiness (T). At the bottom of the worksheet, the partners record the changes in emotions and behaviors (C) that emanate from using the most balanced of the thoughts and plan for how the new thoughts, feelings, and

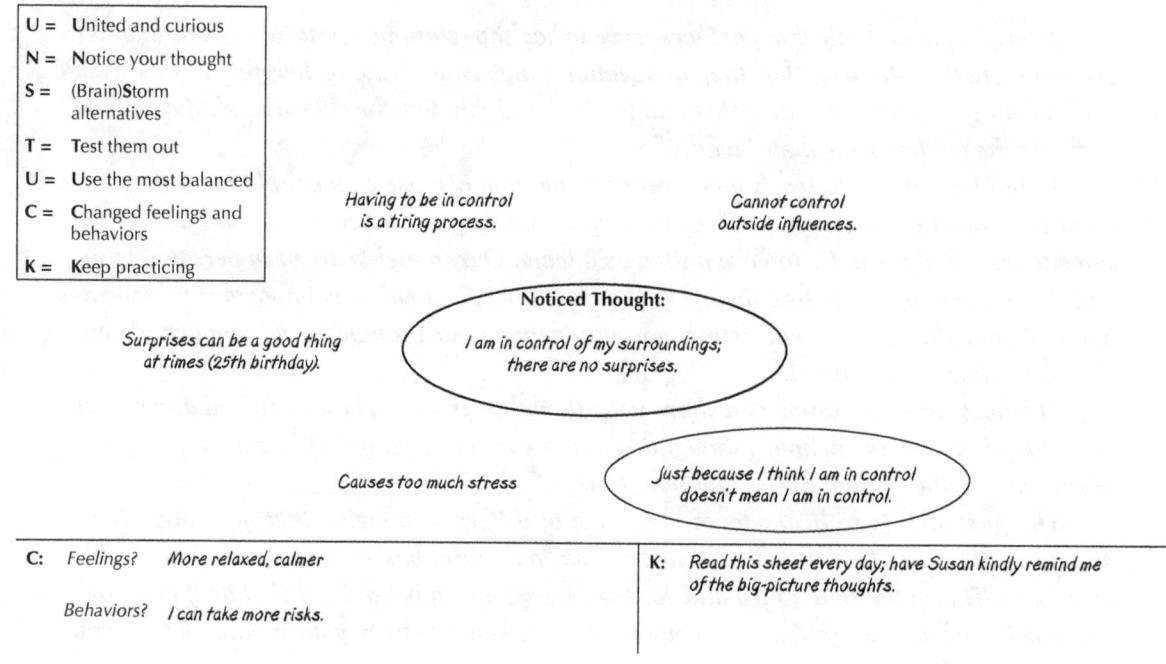

**FIGURE 6.1.** Completed Big Picture worksheet.

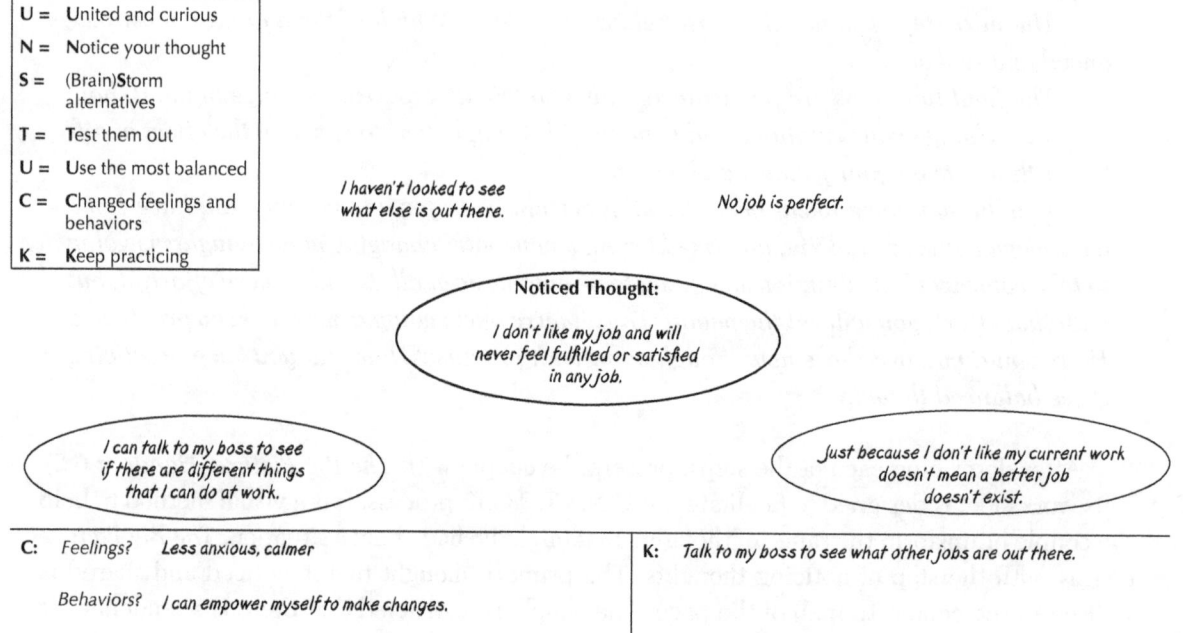

**FIGURE 6.2.** Completed Big Picture worksheet.

Session 6. Getting U.N.S.T.U.C.K.

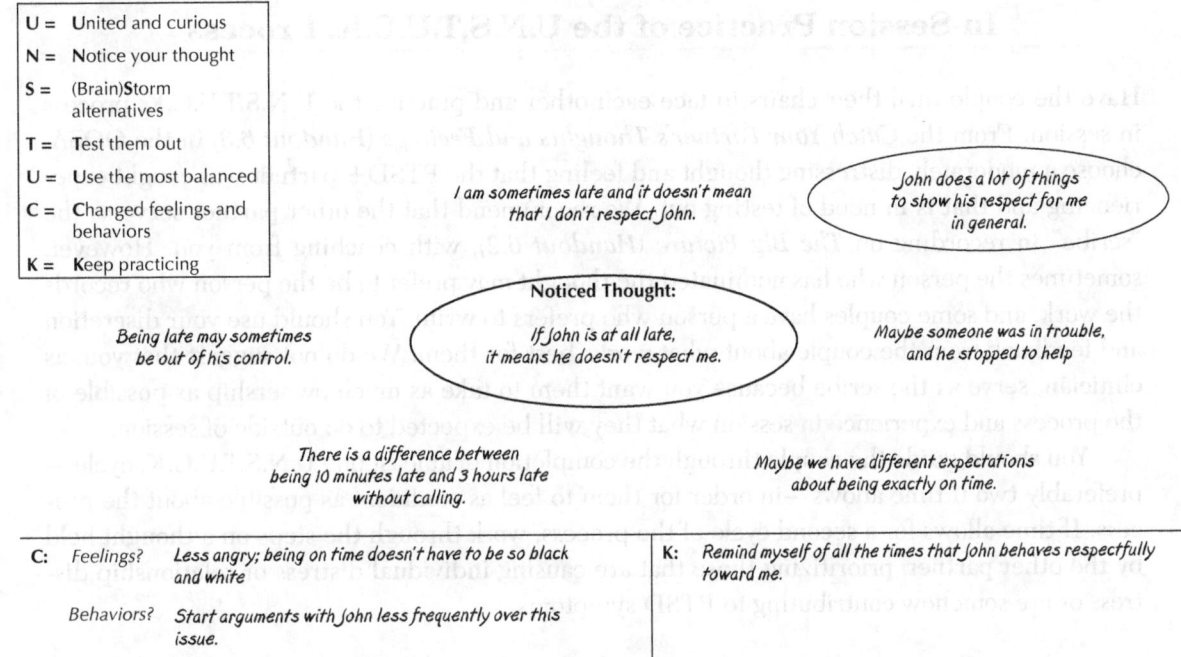

**FIGURE 6.3.** Completed Big Picture worksheet.

behaviors will be practiced and tested (**K**). This worksheet will be used throughout the rest of the therapy. Several examples of successfully completed worksheets are included in Figures 6.1, 6.2, and 6.3.

> To help you in the U.N.S.T.U.C.K. process, we have a worksheet called *The Big Picture*, a visual means for the two of you to consider the possibility that tunnel-vision thinking may be occurring. All of us can narrow our "vision" to see things in a certain way. You've probably heard people talk about tunnel vision. When we have tunnel vision, we can't see the big picture and other possible explanations. This sheet is designed to help you consider the big picture, or panoramic, way of thinking about a situation.
>
> You will record the primary thought that is noticed in the center. The space outside of the circle is designed for you to record alternative thoughts, the **S** step of (brain)storming alternative thoughts. Both of you will offer thoughts to write outside of the "bubble." This form will be a sort of "table" upon which you can place your thoughts to test them together, the **T** step. We recommend that you circle the balanced or most effective thought or thoughts in the **U** step to help you focus on them.
>
> Steps **C** and **K** are included at the bottom of the page as a place for you to record how the balanced thoughts make you feel and how you predict you will act (**C**) and for you to describe ways that you will keep practicing and testing these thoughts. Examples of what you might do to keep practicing include reading over *The Big Picture* on a regular basis, placing it where you see it often, or developing some plan to test out the new belief (e.g., ask a person whom you are "mind reading" what he or she actually thinks about a situation).

## In-Session Practice of the U.N.S.T.U.C.K. Process

Have the couple turn their chairs to face each other and practice the U.N.S.T.U.C.K. process in session. From the *Catch Your Partner's Thoughts and Feelings* (*Handout 6.3*) in the OOSA, choose a moderately distressing thought and feeling that the PTSD+ partner was caught experiencing and that is in need of testing out. We recommend that the other partner serve as the "scribe" in recording on *The Big Picture* (*Handout 6.2*), with coaching from you. However, sometimes the person who has nominated the thought may prefer to be the person who records the work, and some couples have a person who prefers to write. You should use your discretion and feedback from the couple about what works best for them. We do not suggest that you, as clinician, serve as the scribe because you want them to take as much ownership as possible of the process and experience in session what they will be expected to do outside of session.

You should guide the couple through the completion of at least one U.N.S.T.U.C.K. cycle—preferably two if time allows—in order for them to feel as confident as possible about the process. If time allows for a second cycle of the process, work through the steps on a thought held by the other partner, prioritizing those that are causing individual distress or relationship distress or are somehow contributing to PTSD symptoms.

## Shrinking PTSD through Approach

From the *Avoidance List* (*Handout 3.2*), determine the next place, situation, thing, or feeling that will be approached prior to the next session. Record the item on the *OOSA summary* (*Handout 6.4*) and ask the couple to write about how it went.

As in previous sessions, anticipate with the couple barriers to the success of carrying out the approach behavior and preemptively problem solve how those behaviors might be overcome. Refer them to the PROUD acronym in *Handout 4.3* to help strategize maximizing the benefits of the approach exercise.

## Out-of-Session Assignments

Orient the couple to the *OOSA summary* (*Handout 6.4*) for this session and point out the following assignments:

- Continue to monitor positive behaviors in each other, even though they will not be asked to record these behaviors on a daily basis.
- Have the couple use the U.N.S.T.U.C.K. process with *The Big Picture* (*Handout 6.2*) at least four times prior to the next session (more if they are willing). The PTSD+ partner should nominate at least one trauma-related cognition and the other partner should nominate any cognitions that he or she is struggling with (trauma related or not). Prioritize partners' stuck points that may impede their own (in dual-PTSD cases) or their partner's (e.g., "My partner being distressed means her PTSD is worse") recovery. Each partner should also nominate a relationship-related cognition that each has.

- Relationship-oriented cognitions that affect relationship satisfaction and functioning often relate to negative attributions about partner behaviors or unrealistic standards applied to the relationship or partner. Some examples include:
  - Her being late means that she has no respect for me. (attribution)
  - He is only with me to gratify his own needs. (attribution)
  - Our decreased sexual activity means that she is interested in someone else. (attribution)
  - He cheated because there's something wrong with me.
  - My partner and I should want to spend all of our free time together. (standard)
  - My partner should know my needs without me having to tell him. (standard)
  - My career should come first because I make more money. (standard)
  - We should agree about most everything. (standard)
- During the session, pay attention to thoughts expressed by each member of the couple that would be helpful for them to work on outside of session. This will help increase adherence and help you to be more targeted in your work with them to resolve PTSD and other mental health symptoms and to improve their relationship. We recommend that you, as therapist, help the couple to generate and record on individual *Big Picture* (*Handout 6.2*) worksheets the specific thoughts that they will work on together outside of the session.
- Continue the *Catch Your Partner's Thoughts and Feelings* (*Handout 6.3*) on a daily basis, with at least one trauma-related entry.
- Remind the couple of the item chosen from the *Avoidance List* (*Handout 3.2*) to be approached prior to the next session and ask them to record how it went.

## Check-Out

Ask the couple how the session was for each of them. Are there any lingering concerns or questions? What do they want to take with them from the session to improve their relationship and PTSD? Infuse hopefulness and predict success in completing the OOSAs as they leave the session.

HANDOUT 6.1

# Getting U.N.S.T.U.C.K.

We have been working toward identifying the differences between thoughts and feelings and understanding how thoughts influence feelings. We are taking it to the next step to learn a process that you can use together to consider how helpful or unhelpful your ways of thinking are.

### U = United and Curious

This process is not designed to point out how the other is "wrong" or to be critical and judgmental of each other. The idea is for each of you to be *curious* with one another and to be a team to determine whether the thoughts have a good basis to them and whether they are helpful.

### N = Notice the Way You Are Thinking

Before you can evaluate thoughts and their related feelings, they first have to be noticed. Use your paraphrasing skills to pinpoint thoughts and feelings, making sure that each of you is on the same page about them. This is very important prior to proceeding to the next step. It is often helpful to "boil down" your thoughts to a primary thought or two.

### S = (Brain)Storm Alternative Thoughts

In this step you want to be as open-minded as possible about all of the types of thoughts that might be had in reaction to an event by brainstorming. Both of you should contribute as many different perspectives as possible. Feel free to come up with what might seem like the wildest possible thoughts at this step. Now is *not* the time to be critical!

### T = Test Them

With a range of thoughts on your joint "table," put them to the test. What is the evidence for each of them? Which are the most balanced?

### U = Use the Most Balanced

Which are the most balanced of the thoughts? Which is the most realistic? Which is the most effective? It will feel awkward at first—like wearing a new pair of shoes. Break it in for at least a trial period. Circle the most balanced one(s) on *The Big Picture* (Handout 6.2).

### C = Changes in Emotion and Behaviors

With that new thought in mind, how would you feel? How do you feel? What would you do differently? What are you doing differently?

### K = Keep Practicing

Changing your mind can sometimes be hard work, especially when you've thought strongly one way for a long time. It won't necessarily be automatic at first, but with practice it will become that way. So keep up that effortful practice! *How can you keep new ways of thinking as "alive" as possible? What can you **do** to test them out?*

---

From *Cognitive-Behavioral Conjoint Therapy for PTSD: Harnessing the Healing Power of Relationships* by Candice M. Monson and Steffany J. Fredman. Copyright 2012 by The Guilford Press. Permission to photocopy this handout is granted to purchasers of this book for personal use only (see copyright page for details).

HANDOUT 6.2

# The Big Picture

**Noticed Thought:**

- **U** = **U**nited and curious
- **N** = **N**otice your thought
- **S** = (Brain)**S**torm alternatives
- **T** = **T**est them out
- **U** = **U**se the most balanced
- **C** = **C**hanged feelings and behaviors
- **K** = **K**eep practicing

C: *Feelings?*

*Behaviors?*

K:

---

From *Cognitive-Behavioral Conjoint Therapy for PTSD: Harnessing the Healing Power of Relationships* by Candice M. Monson and Steffany J. Fredman. Copyright 2012 by The Guilford Press. Permission to photocopy this handout is granted to purchasers of this book for personal use only (see copyright page for details).

HANDOUT 6.3

# Catch Your Partner's Thoughts and Feelings

Week of: _____

| | Partner: _____ | | | Partner: _____ | | |
|---|---|---|---|---|---|---|
| | Event | Thought | Feeling | Event | Thought | Feeling |
| Example: | Hear a noise outside | "Someone is trying to break in." | Afraid | Partner brings breakfast in bed. | "My partner cares about me." | Content |
| Sunday | | | | | | |
| Monday | | | | | | |
| Tuesday | | | | | | |
| Wednesday | | | | | | |
| Thursday | | | | | | |
| Friday | | | | | | |
| Saturday | | | | | | |

From *Cognitive-Behavioral Conjoint Therapy for PTSD: Harnessing the Healing Power of Relationships* by Candice M. Monson and Steffany J. Fredman. Copyright 2012 by The Guilford Press. Permission to photocopy this handout is granted to purchasers of this book for personal use only (see copyright page for details).

HANDOUT 6.4

# Out-of-Session Assignments
## Session 6. Getting U.N.S.T.U.C.K.

1. Continue to watch for, and point out, positive behaviors in each other.
2. Use the U.N.S.T.U.C.K. process together at least four times prior to the next session. Practice the process on thoughts that each of you identified on *Catch Your Partner's Thoughts and Feelings* (*Handout 6.3*). You should each work on two thoughts, one individually oriented and one relationship related. At least one of the individually oriented thoughts should be trauma related.
3. Continue to catch each other's thoughts and feelings on a daily basis using *Catch Your Partner's Thoughts and Feelings* (*Handout 6.3*). At least one of the thoughts should be trauma related.
4. Shrinking PTSD through Approach:

_____
(people, place, situation, feeling)

Write about how it went:
_____
_____

Place this form somewhere that is convenient and visible to the two of you.

**Next appointment:** _____ @ _____

---

From *Cognitive-Behavioral Conjoint Therapy for PTSD: Harnessing the Healing Power of Relationships* by Candice M. Monson and Steffany J. Fredman. Copyright 2012 by The Guilford Press. Permission to photocopy this handout is granted to purchasers of this book for personal use only (see copyright page for details).

# SESSION 7

# Problem Solving to Shrink PTSD

> ### SUMMARY OF SESSION CONTENT
>
> #### Goals
>
> - Teach problem-solving/decision-making skills. These skills are recommended to be used after something is accurately determined to be a problem or when a decision needs to be made, either through the U.N.S.T.U.C.K. process or through good sharing thoughts and feelings skills.
> - Help the couple learn a process whereby they can make decisions about how they, as a couple, can work together to shrink the role of PTSD in their relationship by (1) improving communication and thereby decreasing conflict and (2) decreasing behavioral avoidance of places or situations that they have continued to avoid.
>
> #### Key Interventions
>
> 1. Review of Out-of-Session Assignments
>    - Notice Positive Behaviors in Each Other
>    - The Big Picture (Handout 6.2)
>    - Catch Your Partner's Thoughts and Feelings (Handout 6.3)
>    - Shrinking PTSD through Approach (Handout 6.4)
> 2. Introduction to Problem Solving/Decision Making (*Problem-Solving/Decision-Making Guidelines, Handout 7.1*)
>    - Introduce the problem-solving/decision-making channel to the couple.
>    - Explain the principles of good problem solving /decision making.
> 3. In-Session Practice/Shrinking PTSD through Approach
>    - The couple uses their problem-solving skills to decide on an *in vivo* approach task.
>    - Start the couple on a second problem on which to use their skills (if time permits).
> 4. Out-of-Session Assignments (*Handout 7.3*)
>    - Notice Positive Behaviors in Each Other
>    - Problem-Solving/Decision-Making Guidelines (Handout 7.1)
>    - Practice Making a Decision Together Using the Guidelines
>    - The Big Picture (Handout 7.2)
>    - Shrinking PTSD through Approach (Handout 7.3)
> 5. Check-Out

**\*Administer the patient and partner versions of PCL/relationship happiness.**

# Review of Out-of-Session Assignments

## Positive Behaviors

Inquire about positive behaviors that the couple has noticed in themselves and their partner.

## The Big Picture (Handout 6.2)

Have the couple explain their use of the U.N.S.T.U.C.K. process on their respective cognitions. It is important that, as a therapist, you are beginning to hand the therapy process over to them more and more as you are now about halfway done with the course of therapy. In this spirit, you should work to become more of an observer of their shared process, coaching them on ways in which the U.N.S.T.U.C.K. procedure and use of *The Big Picture* worksheet was not optimized.

If you have had adequate OOSA compliance to this point, it is unlikely that the couple will not have completed the U.N.S.T.U.C.K. process on their cognitions prior to the session. However, if they did not complete the process, ask questions to determine whether there is a problem in understanding the tool or a motivational issue in using it. This understanding will help you to intervene most effectively. Psychoeducation should be used if there is a knowledge deficit. We recommend Socratic dialogue if there appears to be a motivational issue (e.g., "What got in the way of your doing the process together?"; "What part(s) felt most difficult to you?"). Some stumbling blocks to anticipate include the following.

## Overidentification with Thoughts

The partner who nominated the thought that is the object of the U.N.S.T.U.C.K. process may feel defensive, possibly believing that his or her thoughts are being critiqued and, therefore, he or she is being criticized. The primary intervention in this case is to objectify the thoughts from the person targeted in the process. In this case, it may be very helpful to use the U.N.S.T.U.C.K. process itself to flesh out and, it is hoped, resolve any ambivalence about the intervention (e.g., primary thought = "testing my thoughts is testing me as a person"). It is helpful to remind partners that they themselves determine their thoughts; their thoughts don't determine them.

## "Attacking" Partner

Sometimes individuals take their role of challenging their partner's thoughts very seriously and can come off too attacking or critical. The primary intervention in this case is to stress the importance of the couple being on the same team, united together to determine the helpfulness of thoughts. We often highlight this softer, more collaborative role, as opposed to one partner's playing the role of a "district attorney" in which he or she tries to wear down the other partner by pointing out holes in his or her logic. Introducing a Socratic dialogue that elicits softer sentiments toward each other—for example, "Is there anything that Pam might do to make you feel safer in the U.N.S.T.U.C.K. process?"—can be helpful.

Another strategy is to unite the couple through externalization of PTSD. As applicable, orient the couple to consider the PTSD as making them think a certain way. In this way, the couple is challenging PTSD and not the individual. For several couples who we have treated, PTSD was described as a little gnome or monster who sat on the PTSD+ partner's shoulder, feeding negative thoughts. We encouraged the couples to "talk back" to the PTSD (not the person with PTSD) with the alternative thoughts that they generated together.

## Changed Thoughts but Not a Change of Heart

This is perhaps *the* most common feedback that couples will provide about the U.N.S.T.U.C.K. process. If it doesn't arise in this session, we can almost guarantee that it will arise at some point in the therapy course. We suggest the following principles in dealing with this feedback:

1. **Validate.** Validate that a change in thoughts is not necessarily going to elicit an immediate change in feelings. Also, validate the couple's open-mindedness and creativity in identifying alternative thoughts. We often congratulate clients that they are halfway to changing their emotions and behavior if they can at least *consider* alternative ways of thinking. For those with a substance abuse history or in a relationship with someone with such a history, it can be helpful to use the analogy that recognition is perhaps the most important step to recovery.

2. **Promote practice.** Changing one's thinking is like learning anything new or changing any other habit: It takes effortful practice. Metaphors that we have successfully used include *sports analogies* (e.g., "When you first learned to swing a golf club or a baseball bat or shoot a basketball, it wasn't rote—you had to think carefully about what you were doing. With time, it becomes more automatic. Have you ever picked up a bad habit in that sport? What did it take to correct that habit?"), *ruts in a road* (e.g., "An automobile can cruise effortlessly down a well-worn road of ruts. But what happens when you try to pull the car out of the ruts? It takes effort. It takes consistent effort to make a new set of ruts that allow the car to cruise down the road"), and *neuroscience* (e.g., "Overlearned thoughts have well-developed synaptic pathways. It takes effort to generate synaptic pathways to new areas of our brains, and sometimes our brains follow old pathways when we're not practicing effortful attention").

3. **Promote hope.** Instill a sense of hope about the future ease in which a person will think in new ways after he or she has put in hard work toward practice. Point out that it is likely difficult for them to imagine the new thought being automatic, but that you (even if using the collective "you") *know* that this will occur based on the experience of prior patients who have received this therapy. We often use the metaphor of children growing to describe the expected subtle changes that will occur. Have you ever been around children enough that you didn't notice that they were growing, but someone who is not around them as much seemed struck by how much they had grown? This more subtle trajectory is the path of most cognitive change. Of course, there are a minority of patients, in our experience, who have epiphanies or flashes of insight, have an immediate cognitive shift, and have experienced relatively immediate positive emotional and behavioral benefits (i.e., sudden gains in the research literature; Kelly, Rizvi, Monson, & Resick, 2009). We find this more frequently with regard to the appraisal of specific events and, in this treatment, the appraisal of traumatic events.

You are also likely to have heard at least one member of the couple say in response to an U.N.S.T.U.C.K. process, "I know what you're saying, but I don't really believe it" or "My head gets it, but my heart doesn't." The important principle is to reinforce the couple for their open-mindedness because getting something cognitively is a fundamental step toward longer standing emotional and behavioral change. There are several avenues that you can pursue when this occurs.

- **Practice.** This might include the couple reading and rehearsing daily a successful *Big Picture* assignment or having the couple agree to have one partner remind the other of the new thought. We often use analogies to help reinforce the notion that a new thought will not feel "natural" or "automatic" at first. Examples include sports analogies involving tennis strokes, golf swings, and football passes. When first using these skills, they are labored and you really have to think about it, but with repetition they become automatic. Other analogies include driving a car into a rut. It takes effort to get the car wheels out of the well-worn rut. Our automatic thoughts are those well-worn ruts, and it takes efforts to make a new, healthier path.

- **Pairing cognitive practice and *in vivo* approach.** We have had success in having couples read over a successful *Big Picture* assignment prior to completing a relevant approach assignment and then debriefing afterward. In this way, the worksheet served as a cognitive reminder or primer, reinforced by testing out the thought behaviorally. This can help strengthen the new thought. The challenge with this technique is finding approach assignments to pair with the U.N.S.T.U.C.K. process.

We once worked with a couple in which one partner avoided taking public transportation because of fears that someone would blow up the bus or subway. As a result of his hypervigilance, he also sat with his back to the wall in restaurants so that he could scan the environment for possible threatening cues. Several times, the couple completed approach assignments that involved their riding the bus and then going to a restaurant and the PTSD+ partner sitting with his back to the door. However, when they described how it had gone, the PTSD+ partner reported that his anxiety had not really decreased during or after the exercise. Further discussion revealed that he had essentially been "white knuckling" his way through the exercise and had continued to fuel his anxiety during the exercise with the thought, "Someone could do something terrorist-like at any time, and I have to be on my guard to stop it." To help him maximally profit from the *in vivo* approach activities, the therapist paired the U.N.S.T.U.C.K. process with the exercise, as follows:

> THERAPIST: Jim, it's great that you went on the bus instead of driving, as you usually do to manage your anxiety, and that you went to the restaurant and sat with your back to the door. I'm curious, though, as to why you think you might not have felt less anxious after doing these things and seeing that nothing bad happened?
>
> JIM: I don't know. I just felt like I couldn't really relax while I was in it.
>
> THERAPIST: Sarah, what questions do you have for Jim about why he couldn't relax?
>
> SARAH: Were you thinking that something bad could still happen?
>
> JIM: Yeah, I think I was.
>
> THERAPIST: So, Jim, if I'm hearing you correctly, it sounds as though you were "white knuckling" your way through it rather than being fully present in the moment and having it feel natural? That sounds like one of those obstacles, or "O," on the PROUD to Shrink PTSD handout.

JIM: Yes, that's right.

THERAPIST: You guys are doing great work so far, and I'd really like to see you benefit fully from all of your efforts. I'm going to propose that you do the U.N.S.T.U.C.K. process before you go out next time so that you can have that new, more balanced thought on your mind and available to you while you're in the situation. That way, I think you'll be able to put your new thinking in action with your approach. What do you think?

SARAH: That makes sense to me.

JIM: Okay, I'll give it a try.

THERAPIST: Great. Let's have you work together to identify the thought that Jim tends to have while on the bus or in a restaurant with his back to the door. (U—United and curious)

JIM: Someone could do something terrorist-like at any time, and I have to be on my guard to stop it. (N—Notice your thought)

SARAH: That's technically true, but how likely is it that that would happen here? (S—(Brain) Storm alternatives)

JIM: It happened a lot in Iraq.

SARAH: Yes, but that was a war zone. What's the actual likelihood that something like that will happen here? (T—testing them out)

JIM: I guess it's less likely.

THERAPIST: Let's really try to "right size" those odds. Jim, what's your best guess as to how likely it is that someone will blow up the bus in Boston in a terrorist act?

JIM: Ten percent.

SARAH: That means one out of 10 times that people ride the bus here in Boston there's a terrorist act that occurs.

JIM: I guess that does seem pretty high. Maybe I'm overestimating. It's probably more like less than 1%.

THERAPIST: That sounds more realistic. Maybe even less? How would you boil down that alternative thought into a sentence?

JIM: We can't say the odds are zero because we can never rule out the random possibility that a terrorist act could happen on the bus, but the odds are probably quite small here in Boston now.

THERAPIST: Do you really believe that new thought?

JIM: When I put it down on paper, it seems pretty obvious (U—Use the most balanced)

THERAPIST: Sarah, what do you think of that new thought?

SARAH: It makes sense to me as I hear it. Jim, how do you feel as you go from the thought "Someone could do something terrorist-like at any time, and I have to be on my guard to stop it" to "Although we can never be 100% sure that something bad won't happen, it's extremely unlikely and the odds are probably close to zero here in Boston"?

JIM: I feel less anxious and on guard. (C—Changed feelings and behaviors)

THERAPIST: Great work. Now, to really have this thought stick, I'd like you to review this work as you've recorded it on your sheet before the next time you get on the bus and go to the restaurant (K—Keep practicing). While you're on the bus and in the restaurant, I'd like you both to keep reminding Jim of this new, more balanced thought until sitting on the bus or eating in the restaurant with your back to the door feels more natural to you. Then, after you come home, I'd like you to talk with each other about how it went. My expectation is that the more you do this and use that new, more balanced thought in the moment, the more it will feel second nature to you.

- **Deeper beliefs.** Sometimes there are deeper, schema-level beliefs that prevent the couple from fully embracing a new way of thinking. It is often helpful to ask, "What part of the new thought is hardest for you to believe?" or "What would it mean if you fully embraced that thought?" The answers can give you clues to the underlying belief. A common example that we encounter relates to acceptance that the traumatized person could not have done something different to prevent the event (i.e., undoing). The conclusion would then be "I can't control everything bad from happening." The work is then to "right-size" the deeper belief to be less extreme, on the order of "I can control many bad things from happening, but certainly not all bad things. Sometimes bad things are beyond my control."

### *Catch Your Partner's Thoughts and Feelings (Handout 6.3)*

Review the couple's responses to this form using the suggestions presented in the prior session.

### *Shrinking PTSD through Approach (Handout 6.4)*

Review how the *in vivo* assignment went and reinforce any approach behavior and couple-level facilitation of such. Troubleshoot ways in which the couple may have accommodated avoidance. If the couple was successful in approaching an item off of the *Avoidance List* (*Handout 3.2*), in some way note this on their list (e.g., cross it out if no longer avoided, place a checkmark if previously assigned but still working on it more).

## Introduction to Problem Solving/Decision Making

To help reinforce the different types of communication that the couple may have, remind them that there are two channels for communication and that we have previously been focused on the channel regarding sharing. In this session, we will be focusing on the channel of problem solving/decision making. It may be helpful to orient them to *Communication Channel* (*Handout 4.1*) from their binder, highlighting the two types of communication.

The last three sessions have been spent on the sharing thoughts and feelings channel to help the couple identify their thoughts and emotions and to share them with each other as one way of shrinking the role of PTSD in their relationship. This type of communication serves as an antidote to emotional/experiential avoidance and fosters emotional intimacy. The current session focuses on the other channel: problem solving/decision making. The goal of this session is to help the couple learn a process whereby they can make decisions about how they, as a couple, can work together to shrink the role of PTSD in their relationship by (1) improving communication and thereby decreasing conflict and (2) decreasing behavioral avoidance of places or situations that they have continued to avoid. This can be especially helpful when partners disagree about whether and how to approach feared situations. It can also help decrease conflict and hyperarousal by helping them strategize how to get both of their needs met when they disagree about something. **It may be helpful to think about the U.N.S.T.U.C.K. process as *cognitive* solving, whereas problem-solving skills taught in this session are about *behavioral* solving.** Common to both strategies is the emphasis on brainstorming and increasing the couple's ability to flexibly consider a range of possible solutions.

The following are some guidelines that can help people make good decisions together as a couple. Emphasize that these are not **rules** but rather **principles** to optimize the chances that they can both get their needs met.

1. Use your listening and paraphrasing skills to ***pinpoint*** clearly and specifically the problem or decision to be made.
2. Use sharing thoughts and feelings to ***clarify why the issue is important and what your needs are***.
3. ***Brainstorm*** possible solutions or decisions without judgment.
4. Decide on a ***solution that is agreeable*** to both of you.
5. Decide on a ***trial period*** to implement the solution.

Give the *Problem-Solving/Decision-Making Guidelines* (*Handout 7.1*) to the couple while you are explaining the principles.

## In-Session Practice/Shrinking PTSD through Approach

Have the couple turn their chairs to face each other to practice using problem-solving/decision-making skills to decide on their next *in vivo* approach assignment. The *in vivo* approach assignment should involve something more difficult than that for the previous week.

It may be tempting to choose a more difficult topic with which to practice the problem-solving/decision-making skills. We recommend against this, at least as the initial topic. You want the couple to have the opportunity to practice the entire set of principles in session with a decision that can be made. If time allows, by all means start the couple on another chosen problem or decision. Even if they do not complete the process in session, they can continue the process outside of session, armed with at least one successful trial of the skills in session.

As in previous sessions, anticipate with the couple barriers to the success of carrying out the approach behavior and preemptively problem solve how those behaviors might be overcome. Refer them to the PROUD acronym in *Handout 4.3* to help strategize maximizing the benefits of the approach exercise.

## Out-of-Session Assignments

Orient the couple to the *OOSA summary sheet* (*Handout 7.3*) for this session and point out the following assignments:

- Continue to monitor positive behaviors in each other, even though they will not be asked to record these behaviors on a daily basis.
- Read over *Problem-Solving/Decision-Making Guidelines* (*Handout 7.1*) together and practice problem solving/decision making on at least two different problems/decisions prior to the next session.
- Have the couple use the U.N.S.T.U.C.K. process with *The Big Picture* (*Handout 7.2*) at least four times prior to the next session (more if they are willing). The PTSD+ partner should nominate at least one trauma-related cognition, and the other partner should nominate any cognitions that he or she is struggling with (trauma related or not). Prioritize partners' stuck points that may impede their own (in dual-PTSD cases) or their partner's recovery (e.g., "My partner being distressed means her PTSD is worse"). Partners should also nominate a relationship-related cognition that each has.

    During the session, pay attention to thoughts expressed by each member of the couple that would be helpful for them to work on outside of session. This will help increase adherence and help you to be more targeted in your work with them to resolve PTSD and other mental health symptoms and to improve their relationship. We recommend that you help the couple to generate and record on individual *Big Picture* (*Handout 7.2*) worksheets the specific thoughts that partners will work on together outside of the session.
- Remind the couple of the item chosen from the *Avoidance List* (*Handout 3.2*) to be approached prior to the next session and ask them to record how it went.

## Check-Out

Ask the couple how the session was for each of them. Do they have any lingering concerns or questions? What do they want to take with them from the session to improve their relationship and PTSD? Infuse hopefulness and predict success in completing the OOSAs as they leave the session.

HANDOUT 7.1

# Problem-Solving/Decision-Making Guidelines

1. Use your listening and paraphrasing skills to **pinpoint** clearly and specifically the problem or decision to be made.

   _____

   _____

2. Use sharing thoughts and feelings to **clarify why the issue is important and what your needs are**.

   _____

   _____

3. **Brainstorm** possible solutions or decisions without judgment.

   _____

   _____

   _____

   _____

   _____

   _____

   _____

   _____

4. Decide on a **solution that is agreeable** to both of you.

   _____

   _____

5. Decide on a **trial period** to implement the solution.

   _____

   _____

---

From *Cognitive-Behavioral Conjoint Therapy for PTSD: Harnessing the Healing Power of Relationships* by Candice M. Monson and Steffany J. Fredman. Copyright 2012 by The Guilford Press. Permission to photocopy this handout is granted to purchasers of this book for personal use only (see copyright page for details).

HANDOUT 7.2

# The Big Picture

Noticed Thought:

C: Feelings?

Behaviors?

K:

- U = United and curious
- N = Notice your thought
- S = (Brain)Storm alternatives
- T = Test them out
- U = Use the most balanced
- C = Changed feelings and behaviors
- K = Keep practicing

From *Cognitive-Behavioral Conjoint Therapy for PTSD: Harnessing the Healing Power of Relationships* by Candice M. Monson and Steffany J. Fredman. Copyright 2012 by The Guilford Press. Permission to photocopy this handout is granted to purchasers of this book for personal use only (see copyright page for details).

HANDOUT 7.3

# Out-of-Session Assignments
## Session 7. Problem Solving to Shrink PTSD

1. Continue to watch for, and point out, positive behaviors in each other.
2. Read over *Problem-Solving/Decision-Making Guidelines* (*Handout 7.1*) together.
3. Practice problem solving/decision making at least **twice** prior to the next session. What were the two topics?
   _____
   _____
4. Use the U.N.S.T.U.C.K process together at least four times prior to the next session. You should each work on two thoughts, one individually oriented and one relationship related. At least one of the individually oriented thoughts should be trauma related.
5. Shrinking PTSD through Approach:
   _____
   (people, place, situation, feeling)

   Write about how it went:
   _____
   _____

Place this form somewhere that is convenient and visible to the two of you.

**Next appointment:** _____ @ _____

---

From *Cognitive-Behavioral Conjoint Therapy for PTSD: Harnessing the Healing Power of Relationships* by Candice M. Monson and Steffany J. Fredman. Copyright 2012 by The Guilford Press. Permission to photocopy this handout is granted to purchasers of this book for personal use only (see copyright page for details).

# PHASE 3

# Making Meaning of the Trauma(s) and End of Therapy

# SESSION 8

# Acceptance

## SUMMARY OF SESSION CONTENT

### Goals

- Promote acceptance of the traumatic event(s) by helping the couple move from a tunnel-vision view of the event(s) to a more fully contextualized, elaborated, and big-picture view.
- Begin generating with the couple a formal list of the potential stuck points (problematic thoughts) that have been maintaining the PTSD and any relationship difficulties. This will help focus the work to be done in the remainder of the therapy.

### Key Interventions

1. Review of Out-of-Session Assignments
   - *Notice Positive Behaviors in Each Other*
   - *Problem-Solving/Decision-Making Guidelines* (Handout 7.1)
   - *Practice Making a Decision Together Using the Guidelines*
   - *The Big Picture* (Handout 7.2)
   - *Shrinking PTSD through Approach* (Handout 7.3)
2. Introduction to Phase 3: Meaning Making
   - Remind the couple of the purpose of the prior skill-building phases of the treatment.
   - Reinforce the couple's mastery of the communication skills.
   - Provide a reminder about trauma disclosure.
3. Introduction to Acceptance (*Barriers to Acceptance*, Handout 8.2)
   - Explain what is meant by the term "acceptance."
   - Review the core cognitive barriers to acceptance.
4. In-Session Practice: *U.N.S.T.U.C.K.* to Promote Acceptance
   - Refer to the couple's TIQ-I (*Handout 1.5*) regarding barriers to acceptance.
   - The couple generates stuck points related to acceptance.
   - Use problem solving/decision making around any issues that arise.
5. Shrinking PTSD through Approach
   - Determine at least one person, place, situation, or feeling to be approached.
   - Record the item on the *OOSA summary* (Handout 8.4).
6. Out-of-Session Assignments (*Handout 8.4*)
   - *Stuck Point List* (Handout 8.1)
   - *Barriers to Acceptance* (Handout 8.2)
   - *The Big Picture* (Handout 8.3)
   - *Communication Skills Practice* (Handout 8.4)
   - *Shrinking PTSD through Approach* (Handout 8.4)
7. Check-Out

*Administer the patient and partner versions of PCL/relationship happiness.

## Review of Out-of-Session Assignments

- *Positive Behaviors.* Inquire about positive behaviors that the couple has noticed in themselves and their partner.

- *Problem Solving/Decision Making Guidelines (Handout 7.1).* Have the couple review with you their use of the problem-solving/decision-making principles. Inquire about what worked or didn't seem to work and fine tune their use of the skill. Remind the couple that this skill will be used in conjunction with the U.N.S.T.U.C.K. process once they have collaboratively determined a realistic, balanced view of the situation.

- *The Big Picture (Handout 7.2).* Have the couple explain their use of the U.N.S.T.U.C.K. process on their respective cognitions. Reinforce the couple's hard work in doing the assignment, troubleshoot what got in the way of completing the assignment, and/or coach them on ways in which the U.N.S.T.U.C.K. procedure and use of *The Big Picture* worksheet could be optimized.

- *Shrinking PTSD through Approach (Handout 7.3).* Review how the *in vivo* assignment went and reinforce any approach behavior and couple-level facilitation of such. Troubleshoot ways in which the couple may have accommodated avoidance. If the couple was successful in approaching an item off of the *Avoidance List (Handout 3.2)*, in some way note this on their list (e.g., cross it out if no longer avoided, place a checkmark if previously assigned but still working on it).

## Introduction to Phase 3: Meaning Making

You should segue out of the review of the OOSAs to introduce the final phase of the therapy, focused on making healthier meaning of traumatic events. It is important to set the stage for this transition by reminding the couple of the purpose of building skills in Phases 1 and 2. The prior skill development will serve as a platform for approaching trauma memories and reappraising the events to facilitate recovery. Remind the couple of the two targets that promote recovery in the therapy (i.e., behavioral interventions to address avoidance and numbing, and cognitive interventions to address problematic meaning making), and point out that they have made tremendous progress in addressing avoidance and emotional numbing heretofore. They have also been developing their skills to understand how their thinking influences how they feel. All of those skills are now used to address specific ways that they have made sense of traumatic events that are getting in the way of recovery.

By now, you should have some idea of the potential thoughts maintaining PTSD and relationship difficulties. We have found it helpful at this point in the therapy to start generating a formal list of these thoughts with the couple to help focus the work to be done in Phase 3 of the treatment (see *Stuck Point List, Handout 8.1*). Sessions 8 and beyond should be particularly rich with thoughts that can be targeted using the U.N.S.T.U.C.K. process.

Aside from the patient's and partner's appraisals about the traumatic event(s) itself that will need to be addressed for recovery, there are also **cognitions that the patient or partner might have about what it means to face the traumatic memory that may be impeding recovery.** An example from our clinical practice is a partner without PTSD who was convinced that facing traumatic material would prompt a heart attack in her PTSD+ partner. As a result, she frequently encouraged him to avoid feared places and situations, which, in turn, compromised the potency of the *in vivo* approach exercises. This class of cognitions and the associated accommodative behaviors need to be a focus of intervention in order for the couple to profit fully from the treatment. Cognitions such as these should be the focus of the U.N.S.T.U.C.K. process.

It is very important to reinforce the improvements the couple has made and their hard work in developing and honing their skills. This is important in infusing a sense of mastery and efficacy to address specific traumatic memories.

*The two of you have been doing an excellent job practicing your communication skills and approaching together instead of avoiding and emotionally numbing. You are also making great progress in using the U.N.S.T.U.C.K. process to help one another test out the most balanced way of looking at things. We are going to use all of these great skills to determine whether there are alternative ways of thinking about the trauma and your relationship.*

*The two of you might also have negative thoughts or concerns about what it will mean to go back to work on your thoughts about the traumatic event(s). Those can be barriers to recovery that we will also want to put out there on the table and submit to the U.N.S.T.U.C.K. process.*

*I have every reason to believe that the two of you together will be able to use your skills to put those thoughts on the table and figure out whether there is a healthier, more balanced way for you to make sense of what happened and what will happen when you approach the past.*

### *Reminder about Trauma Disclosure*

It will likely be useful to remind the couple of your stance regarding the disclosure of details of traumatic events. As mentioned, the cognitive theory underlying CBCT for PTSD does not call for nitty-gritty details to increase anxiety for habituation purposes. That said, good Socratic dialogue and consideration of appraisals will necessitate disclosure of some details of events. The details typically elicited involve discussing the chain of events that occurred in order to put things back into their proper perspective. **The Socratic dialogue should not involve eliciting specific details of horrific or grotesque sensory experiences.**

## Introduction to Acceptance

Give *Barriers to Acceptance* (*Handout 8.2*) to the couple and begin reviewing the core cognitive barriers to the acceptance of traumatic events and thereby to recovery. A key concept to be imparted to the couple is that the use of the term "acceptance" in this therapy *does not* imply judgment about the morality or rightfulness of the event or the people involved. Acceptance in this context means not undoing the event, a common cognitive barrier to recovery. As stated in the handout, the event cannot be changed, but one's thoughts and reactions to it can. Your key goal, as the couple's therapist, is to help the PTSD+ person(s) **accept the reality** of the event by putting it back into its **proper context**.

Point out to the couple that most people with PTSD are so avoidant or "phobic" of their trauma memory that they never stop to do a fine-grained analysis to determine why things really happened the way they did and what the event means to them and about them. This is key to developing a better relationship to the memory. The memory will always be there, but they can be more at peace with it. In addition, by sharing one's experiences with others, it makes significant others feel closer, more empathic, and more understanding of the effects of the experience on the person.

Begin walking the couple through the specific cognitive barriers identified in *Barriers to Acceptance* (*Handout 8.2*) as they pertain to retrospection on traumatic events. Following are tips to helping the couple understand the cognitive tendencies:

*When we use the term "acceptance" here, we do **not** mean moral agreement with what happened or condoning the actions of the persons involved. We use "acceptance" here to mean fully coming to terms with the idea that the event happened just the way that it did—accepting that there is nothing that you can do now to change it.*

*An analogy that comes from this therapy is your use of paraphrasing. Just like when you paraphrase each other's comments, you do not necessarily **agree** with the other's position but rather are seeking to hear and understand more fully what the person is saying. We do not expect nor necessarily want you to agree with what happened during the traumatic event, but we do want you to more fully understand, without trying to change, what occurred.*

*With regard to **just-world thinking**, it makes sense to teach this way of thinking to children through school, through religion, and at home, because we don't want kids growing up thinking that negative actions may or may not have negative consequences. However, as we get older, our thinking grows more complex to incorporate the idea that good behaviors don't **always** get rewarded and bad behavior doesn't always get punished. You may think, "A bad thing happened to me. Therefore, I must be a bad person." One other way that just-world thinking can get you in trouble is if you did a "bad" thing. If you say to yourself, "I did a bad thing, so I must be a _____ person," you may not be fully seeing the big picture of everything that was going on at the time that influenced your behavior. That is part of our neglecting situational demands on us at the time of our choices, and we'll talk about this further shortly. This is another reason why we need to take a careful look at what happened in the past to make sure that you're thinking about it in a balanced and realistic way.*

***Undoing** is what we do with our just-world thinking and hindsight biases—we may try to think of all kinds of alternative courses of action that we believe could have prevented a bad outcome. If there would have been a good outcome, do you think you would* be thinking of alternative actions? It is tempting to want to assume that there must have been some way to avoid the negative outcome. The assumption is that if we could just "undo" a choice or choices, the outcome would be different. That assumption may or may not be true.

Part of undoing is the belief that an alternative course of action would have led to a positive outcome—**happily-ever-after or fairytale thinking**. Rarely do people appreciate that another course of action could have led to equally bad or even worse outcomes.

We often think or want to think that we're more powerful than the situation that surrounds us—**situational neglect**. Years of research tells us that the situation is usually more important than the individual in the situation (e.g., Nazi Germany; Haney, Banks, & Zimbardo, 1973; Milgram, 1974). That means that we can sometimes neglect the power of a situation when we make decisions. Examples include remembering the consequences that would ensue if a command was disobeyed, the peer pressure imposed by those around you, the knife, the gun or other weapon in the situation, and so on. These are important variables that must be fully appreciated when seeing the big picture of the situation.

The completed *Big Picture* worksheet in Figure 8.1 illustrates types of tunnel-vision thinking that get in the way of accepting the facts of the event as well as thoughts about the entire picture of what happened.

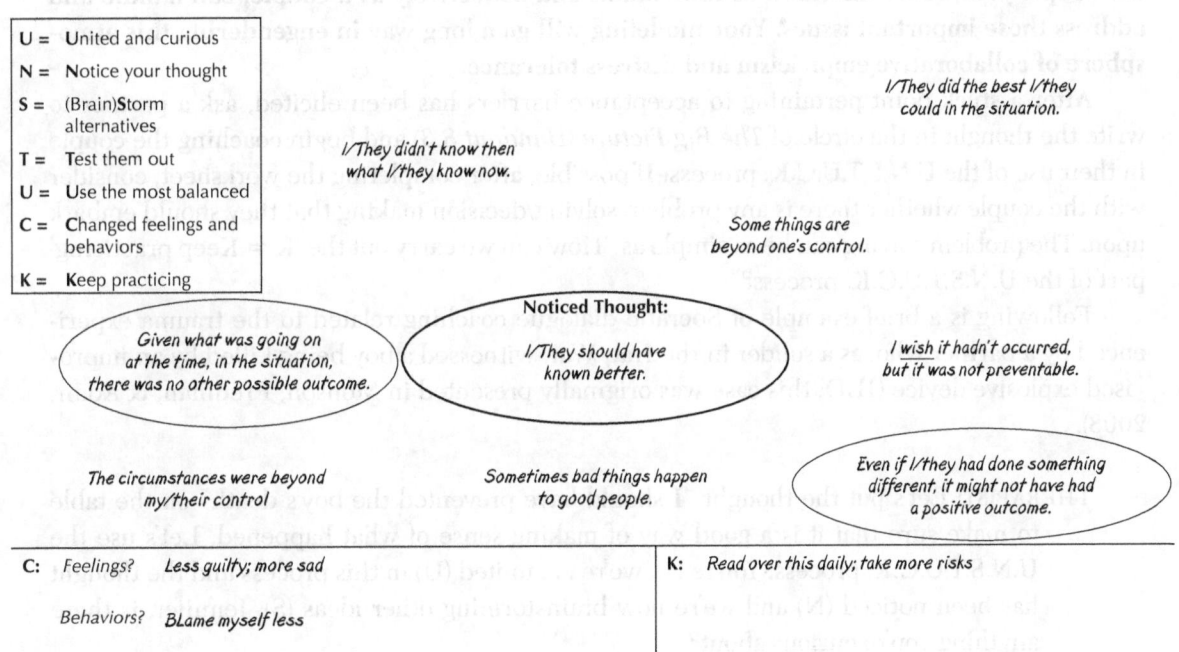

**FIGURE 8.1.** Completed Big Picture worksheet.

## In-Session Practice: U.N.S.T.U.C.K. to Promote Acceptance

After this portion of the psychoeducation is completed, refer back to responses on the TIQ-I (*Handout 1.5*) pertaining to the question about why the traumatic event occurred. You can share these with the couple as additional information about barriers to acceptance of the traumatic event. **Again, the key is to find any ways in which the PTSD+ individual and his or her partner may be trying to deny the reality of the event as it occurred at the time.** Have the couple turn their chairs to face each other to use the U.N.S.T.U.C.K. process to begin to address stuck points related to acceptance of the traumatic event. In determining the stuck points to work on in this area, it is helpful to listen closely to the PTSD+ partner's reactions to the cognitive barriers to acceptance. When he or she hears about the different types, and as you solicit examples, the PTSD+ partner will often make comments about the specific barriers in his or her own rendition of events. You can also pose questions such as:

- What aspect of the event(s) do you most want to "undo" or change?
- Which part(s) are most difficult for you to accept?
- Are there parts that you blame yourself for?
- Are there parts that you blame others for?
- What do you think you would have, could have, or should have done differently?

**It is incredibly important to maintain a sense of curiosity and to ask and prompt partners to ask lots of questions in a matter-of-fact way. This models openness and conveys to the couple your belief that they, as individuals and collectively as a couple, can handle and address these important issues. Your modeling will go a long way in engendering this atmosphere of collaborative empiricism and distress tolerance.**

After a stuck point pertaining to acceptance barriers has been elicited, ask a partner to write the thought in the circle of *The Big Picture* (*Handout 8.3*) and begin coaching the couple in their use of the U.N.S.T.U.C.K. process. If possible, after completing the worksheet, consider with the couple whether there is any problem solving/decision making that they should embark upon. The problem solving can be as simple as "How can we carry out the 'K = Keep practicing' part of the U.N.S.T.U.C.K. process?"

Following is a brief example of Socratic dialogue coaching related to the trauma experienced by a partner who, as a solider in the Iraq War, witnessed a boy being killed by an improvised explosive device (IED; this case was originally presented in Monson, Fredman, & Adair, 2008).

THERAPIST: Let's put the thought "I should have prevented the boy's death" on the table to make sure that it is a good way of making sense of what happened. Let's use the U.N.S.T.U.C.K. process. You're . . . we're . . . united (U) in this process and the thought has been noticed (N) and we're now brainstorming other ideas (S). Jennifer, is there anything you're curious about?

JENNIFER: Yeah, based on what you've told us, John, I'm curious how you could have prevented it.

JOHN: I could have stopped the boy from running toward it.

JENNIFER: Wasn't he running toward it when you arrived?

JOHN: Yeah, but I could have stopped him.

THERAPIST: *(wanting to highlight hindsight bias)* I'm curious about something, John. Do you mind educating Jennifer and me about one thing? Did you or your friends know at the time that the boy was running toward an IED?

JOHN: *(pause)* No . . . no. But we should have known it was an IED.

THERAPIST: Jennifer, do you have a question for John about that?

JENNIFER: Why should or how could you have known?

JOHN: I don't know. I just should have known *(more angrily)*.

THERAPIST: Okay. Do you mind if I tweak your language a little bit? Is one of the possible alternative thoughts "I *wish* I had known it was an IED, but I didn't at the time?" What do you guys think of that?

JENNIFER: That seems to fit more.

THERAPIST: *(pause)* John, what do you think?

JOHN: Yeah. That's true. *(Softens.)*

THERAPIST: I think this is a good example of the Monday morning quarterbacking you mentioned. It seems like at the time you and your fellow soldiers didn't know that it was an IED. *(pause)* Do the two of you think that "I wish that I/John knew that it was an IED" is a more accurate thought, given the circumstances at the time for John?" (T—testing alternative thoughts)

UNISON: Yeah.

THERAPIST: Let's go through the rest of the steps.

Following is an example of the therapist coaching Susan and Jake, presented in Chapter 2, in Socratic dialogue related to Susan's self-blame regarding the rape:

THERAPIST: It sounds like you believe it's your fault that you were raped. Let's use the U.N.S.T.U.C.K. process to put the thought "I let him rape me" on the table. Susan and Jake, you're united (U) in the process of figuring this out together, and you've noticed the thought "I let him rape me" (N). Now we're going to start considering other ideas and brainstorming alternative ways of looking at the situation (S). Jake, what questions do you have for Susan?

JAKE: What leads you to think that you let him rape you?

SUSAN: Because when I realized what was happening, I froze up and didn't fight back.

JAKE: Yeah, but wasn't he bigger than you? He was a 200-pound athlete and you weighed no more than 120 pounds.

SUSAN: Yeah, but I could have scratched him or punched him or something. Anything—instead of just lying there. It was like I was saying it was okay.

JAKE: Being pinned down and having your clothes pulled off means that you wanted him to do it?

SUSAN: It doesn't matter. I should have screamed, cried for help. I didn't say anything and I just let it happen.

THERAPIST: (*wanting to highlight situational neglect*) Susan, can you tell Jake and me what was going through your mind when this was happening?

SUSAN: (*pause*) I thought he was going to kill me.

THERAPIST: (*pause*) Jake, what questions might you have for Susan, knowing that she thought she would be killed?

JAKE: If you thought he was going to kill you, it would make sense to try to just get through it and not make him angrier by fighting. Do you think it could have been worse if you fought back?

SUSAN: I hadn't thought about it that way. But I just hate that I kind of froze up and felt totally helpless to do anything.

THERAPIST: Susan, do you remember when we talked in the first session about the freeze response? That, in addition to the fight-or-flight response, sometimes people freeze when facing a life-threatening situation because there's nothing they can do to stop it?

SUSAN: Yeah, I remember that.

JAKE: Me too. So are you saying that it was actually a survival mechanism that kicked in for her in that moment and actually probably kept her safer given that this guy was bigger and stronger and had acted like he would kill her if she didn't do what he wanted?

THERAPIST: Yes, that's what I'm proposing we might want to put on the table as an alternative to the thought "I let him rape me." Susan, what do you think of that? (T—testing alternative thoughts)

SUSAN: I'd never thought of it that way before.

THERAPIST: (*highlighting situational neglect*) It seems like at the time there were a lot of things going on that contributed to the way the event played out that were beyond your control. Jake, can you ask Susan what she's thinking right now?

JAKE: What are you thinking as we're talking about this?

SUSAN: That even though I wish I could have prevented him from raping me, there was nothing I could have done differently. He was bigger and stronger, he said he'd kill me if I didn't do what he wanted, and then I froze because I felt totally helpless. As we're talking, I'm also realizing that I had no way of knowing that he was going to do this because we'd hung out a bunch of other times in a friendly way and nothing like this had ever happened before.

JAKE: Yeah, he had the element of surprise on his side.

THERAPIST: So if we were going to boil all this down, what do you think the alternative thought to "I let him rape me" might be?

SUSAN: I wish I hadn't been raped but given the circumstances at the time, there was nothing I could do to prevent it.

JAKE: I'm sorry that you went through that.

SUSAN: Me too.

THERAPIST: And so am I. It's really important that we're now putting everything back in its proper place as it unfolded at the time. Let's go through the rest of the steps to see how you feel as we keep working through this.

Monitor for other stuck points that have emerged during this session and prior sessions that are acceptance oriented. They should be identified and written on the Stuck Point List (*Handout 8.1*) for future work in and out of session. The more stuck points that can be identified in session with the couple, the more likely it is that they can be effectively addressed out of session.

## Shrinking PTSD through Approach

From the *Avoidance List* (*Handout 3.2*), determine the next person, place, situation, or feeling that will be approached prior to the next session. Record the item on the *OOSA summary* (*Handout 8.4*) and ask the couple to write about how it went.

As in previous sessions, anticipate with the couple barriers to the success of carrying out the approach behavior and preemptively problem solve how those behaviors might be overcome. Refer them to the PROUD acronym in *Handout 4.3* to help strategize maximizing the benefits of the approach exercise.

## Out-of-Session Assignments

Orient the couple to the *OOSA summary* (*Handout 8.4*) for this session and point out the following assignments:

- Write any identified stuck points on their *Stuck Point List* (*Handout 8.1*).
- Together, read *Barriers to Acceptance* (*Handout 8.2*).
- Have the couple use the U.N.S.T.U.C.K. process with *The Big Picture* (*Handout 8.3*) at least four times prior to the next session (more if they are willing). The PTSD+ partner should nominate at least one trauma-related cognition, and the other partner should nominate any cognitions that he or she is struggling with (trauma related or not). Prioritize partners' stuck points that may impede their own (in dual-PTSD cases) or their partner's recovery (e.g., "My partner being distressed means her PTSD is worse"). Each partner should also nominate a relationship-related cognition that each has.

    During the session, pay attention to thoughts expressed by each partner that would be helpful for them to work on outside of session. This will help increase adherence and help you to be more targeted in your work with them to resolve PTSD and other mental health symptoms and to improve their relationship. We recommend that you help the couple to generate and record on individual *Big Picture* (*Handout 8.3*) worksheets the specific thoughts that they will work on together outside of the session as well as any identified stuck points on their *Stuck Point List* (*Handout 8.1*).

- Ask the couple to spend 5 minutes each day using their best communication skills with one another (*Handout 8.4*). Explain to them that it is important to keep practicing the communication skills that they have developed; using them every day will help them understand each other's perspectives, bring them closer together, and increase the positivity in their relationship. The more they use these skills, the more the skills will feel natural and will trickle into their everyday conversations. Skills to practice include paraphrasing, channel checking, sharing thoughts and feelings, and catching each other's thoughts and feelings. To complete this assignment every day, they may find it helpful to "schedule" their 5 minutes by prompting their partner: for example, "Can we do our 5 minutes of communication skills practice over dinner at 6 P.M.?"
- Remind the couple of the item chosen from the *Avoidance List* (*Handout 3.2*) that will be approached prior to the next session and ask them to record how it went.

## Check-Out

Ask the couple how the session was for each of them. Are there any lingering concerns or questions? What do they want to take with them from the session to improve their relationship and PTSD? Infuse hopefulness and predict success in completing the OOSAs as they leave the session.

# HANDOUT 8.1
# Stuck Point List

**Stuck Point** | **Balanced Thought**

☐ **Example:** *I'm never safe when I go outside of my home.*

☐

☐

☐

☐

☐

☐

☐

☐

---

From *Cognitive-Behavioral Conjoint Therapy for PTSD: Harnessing the Healing Power of Relationships* by Candice M. Monson and Steffany J. Fredman. Copyright 2012 by The Guilford Press. Permission to photocopy this handout is granted to purchasers of this book for personal use only (see copyright page for details).

HANDOUT 8.2

# Barriers to Acceptance

Most people with PTSD have some part of the traumatic event(s) that is hard for them to accept to have happened. One of the ingredients to getting unstuck and recovering from the event is to **accept that the event happened just as it did**. History cannot be rewritten, but your reactions and understanding of that history can change. An important note: Acceptance of the event *does not* mean that what happened is "right," just, or fair. Rather, the goal is to accept that you cannot change the past and appreciate the full picture outside of your tunnel vision of the event.

**Several types of tunnel vision get in the way of acceptance, including:**

- *Just-world thinking*. "Good things happen to good people. Bad things happen to bad people. A bad thing happened. Thus, I or someone else must have done something wrong."
- *Hindsight bias*. Looking back on a situation, you assume that you have the knowledge *then* that you have *now*. This is also called "Monday morning quarterbacking." Sometimes people also say, "Hindsight is 20/20," meaning that you can see with accuracy after the fact things that you could not see at the time.
- *Undoing*. This involves playing out the event with alternative courses of actions that you believe could have prevented it. Example statements are "If I only would have . . . " or "I should have . . ." or "I could have . . ." or "They should have . . ."
- *Happily-ever-after thinking*. This reflection assumes that a different course of action would have led to a positive outcome.
- *Situational neglect*. A human tendency is to overestimate our own influence on situations, neglecting the powerful situational forces that impact on our and others' choices and behavior.

Many people with PTSD have trouble accepting events because they want to maintain their belief that they or others have complete control over themselves and situations in the past and into the future. The key to getting unstuck is to stop avoiding the memory of the event and to fully appreciate the **entire** picture or context of the situation.

---

From *Cognitive-Behavioral Conjoint Therapy for PTSD: Harnessing the Healing Power of Relationships* by Candice M. Monson and Steffany J. Fredman. Copyright 2012 by The Guilford Press. Permission to photocopy this handout is granted to purchasers of this book for personal use only (see copyright page for details).

HANDOUT 8.3

# The Big Picture

**Noticed Thought:**

C: Feelings?

Behaviors?

K:

---

U = United and curious
N = Notice your thought
S = (Brain)Storm alternatives
T = Test them out
U = Use the most balanced
C = Changed feelings and behaviors
K = Keep practicing

---

From *Cognitive-Behavioral Conjoint Therapy for PTSD: Harnessing the Healing Power of Relationships* by Candice M. Monson and Steffany J. Fredman. Copyright 2012 by The Guilford Press. Permission to photocopy this handout is granted to purchasers of this book for personal use only (see copyright page for details).

163

HANDOUT 8.4

# Out-of-Session Assignments
## Session 8. Getting U.N.S.T.U.C.K. to Promote Acceptance

1. Write any stuck points noticed on the *Stuck Point List* (*Handout 8.1*).
2. Together read *Barriers to Acceptance* (*Handout 8.2*).
3. Use the U.N.S.T.U.C.K. process together at least four times prior to the next session. You should each work on two thoughts, one individually oriented and one relationship related, which can be drawn from the *Stuck Point List* (*Handout 8.1*). At least one of the individually oriented thoughts should be trauma related.
4. Spend 5 minutes each day using your best communication skills with one another. Place a checkmark below for each day you practiced.

| Sunday | Monday | Tuesday | Wednesday | Thursday | Friday | Saturday |
|--------|--------|---------|-----------|----------|--------|----------|
|        |        |         |           |          |        |          |

5. Shrinking PTSD through Approach:

   _____
   (people, place, situation, feeling)

   Write about how it went:
   _____
   _____

**Next appointment:** _____ @ _____

---

From *Cognitive-Behavioral Conjoint Therapy for PTSD: Harnessing the Healing Power of Relationships* by Candice M. Monson and Steffany J. Fredman. Copyright 2012 by The Guilford Press. Permission to photocopy this handout is granted to purchasers of this book for personal use only (see copyright page for details).

# SESSION 9

# Blame

---

### SUMMARY OF SESSION CONTENT

#### Goals
- Provide the couple psychoeducation about the determination and placement of blame.
- Assist the couple in fully appreciating the context of the situation of the traumatic event(s), including the intentions and state of mind of those involved.
- Help the couple determine whether blame, of themselves or others, is appropriate as it relates to the traumatic situation.
- Determine whether forgiveness of self or others is appropriate. This should be determined after effective reappraisal and contextualizing of the traumatic event(s).

#### Key Interventions
1. Review of Out-of-Session Assignments
   - *Stuck Point List* (Handout 8.1)
   - *Barriers to Acceptance* (Handout 8.2)
   - *The Big Picture* (Handout 8.3)
   - *Communication Skills Practice* (Handout 8.4)
   - *Shrinking PTSD through Approach* (Handout 8.4)
2. Introduction to Blame (*Getting U.N.S.T.U.C.K. Regarding Blame*, Handout 9.1)
   - Intentionality/state of mind.
   - Situational context.
   - Forgiveness.
3. In-Session Practice: U.N.S.T.U.C.K. Regarding Blame and Other Stuck Points
   - Refer to the couple's TIQ-I (Handout 1.5) regarding barriers to blame.
   - The couple generates stuck points related to acceptance.
   - Use problem solving/decision making around any issues that arise.
4. Shrinking PTSD through Approach
   - Determine at least one person, place, situation, or feeling to be approached.
   - Record the item on the *OOSA summary* (Handout 9.3).
5. Out-of-Session Assignments (Handout 9.3)
   - *Getting U.N.S.T.U.C.K. Regarding Blame* (Handout 9.1)
   - *The Big Picture* (Handout 9.2)
   - *Communication Skills Practice* (Handout 9.3)
   - *Shrinking PTSD through Approach* (Handout 9.3)
6. Check-Out

*Administer the patient and partner versions of PCL/relationship happiness.

## Review of Out-of-Session Assignments

• *Stuck Point List* (*Handout 8.1*). Notice whether the couple has added any new stuck points to their list or whether there has been progress toward addressing those stuck points previously identified.

• *Barriers to Acceptance* (*Handout 8.2*). Inquire whether either partner had any questions about this handout.

• *The Big Picture* (*Handout 8.3*). Have the couple explain their use of the U.N.S.T.U.C.K. process on their respective cognitions. Reinforce the couple's hard work in doing the assignment, troubleshoot what got in the way of completing the assignment, and/or coach the couple on ways in which the U.N.S.T.U.C.K. procedure and use of *The Big Picture* sheet could be optimized.

• *Communication Skills Practice* (*Handout 8.4*). Inquire about their use of good communication skills since the last session.

• *Shrinking PTSD through Approach* (*Handout 8.4*). Review how the *in vivo* assignment went and reinforce any approach behavior and couple-level facilitation of such. Troubleshoot ways in which the couple may have accommodated avoidance. If the couple was successful in approaching an item off of the *Avoidance List* (*Handout 3.2*), in some way note this on their list (e.g., cross it out if no longer avoided, place a checkmark if previously assigned but still working on it).

## Introduction to Blame

You can usually segue out of the review of an U.N.S.T.U.C.K. exercise about acceptance of traumatic events with ease into psychoeducation about the role of self- and other-blame in traumatic events. As a culture, we are prone to want to ascribe fault to someone when something bad happens, whether it be ourselves or someone else. And sometimes someone *is* to blame for something bad happening. However, sometimes bad things just happen without it being someone's fault. The work of this session, as in Session 8, is to appreciate fully the context of the situation, including the intentions and state of mind of those involved. Readers interested in more theory and research regarding the role of intentionality in causal attributions can consult Joseph (1999) and Shaver and Drown (1986).

Ascribing blame can be another way in which people are not accepting the traumatic event. Inappropriate or misplaced blame can serve as a method of asserting mental control when actual control was not possible in the situation. By blaming oneself or someone else, there is the implication that something could have been done by someone to prevent the event(s). In this way, placing blame can be a way of undoing the event and, consequently, not accepting the event to have occurred just the way that it did.

It is very helpful to encourage both partners to use the term "blame" judiciously because it is fraught with many negative connotations and judgment. The client may be responsible for the client's action or inaction during an event(s) but may not necessarily be at fault or to blame for the consequences. Sometimes there is responsibility without blame per se because the person did not intend to do harm. These examples often involve negligence. Examples might include someone who doesn't adequately care for his or her car and causes an automobile accident, being intoxicated during a firefight or while driving, or not wearing one's seat belt and being involved in a motor vehicle accident. **A crucial element in ascribing blame in our model is determining the traumatized person's state of mind or the state of mind of others at the time of the event.** Two important things to carefully evaluate when determining whether and where blame should be placed are (1) intentionality and state of mind and (2) situational demands impinging on the persons at the time. We consider each in turn.

## *Intentionality/State of Mind*

- A person's intention and state of mind at the time of the event(s) are crucial to evaluating blame. If a person had no intention of harm or negative consequences, then blame is not appropriate. Often, the intentional desire at the time is a positive outcome, but because there is a negative outcome, the backward logic is that he or she did something wrong and is to blame. An example of this inappropriately placed self-blame comes from a case in which a military service member shot a pregnant Iraqi woman and her son after trying unsuccessfully to get them to stop at a checkpoint. His *intention* at the time was to do the opposite of shooting a pregnant woman and her son. In effect, he was trying to *prevent* having to shoot the woman and her son.

- Sometimes blame is inappropriately placed. Take, for example, the childhood sexual abuse victim who blames himself for not ending the abuse. In this case, the blame is inappropriately placed on the victim; the perpetrator had the intention and responsibility for having sex with a minor. It was not the intention of the victim to be sexually abused. To process the trauma fully, the victim needs to appreciate the situational context that prevented him from disclosing, fighting back, and so on (e.g., perpetrator's threats to hurt the victim or other family members if there is disclosure, fear of further physical harm if the child fought back). Another example of inappropriately placed blame can be when others, often authority figures, are blamed for bad outcomes. For example, a service member may blame his commanding officer for the death of a fellow service member when, in fact, the commanding officer was following orders from a superior or made the best decision he could have given the information available to him at the time. If the other person in the situation had good intentions that happened to lead to bad outcomes, then blame should not be placed upon that person. A take-home message is that the best laid plans do not always lead to the best outcomes.

- In the case of combat, an appropriate placement of blame that is sometimes overlooked is the enemy. The "best" enemy can foil the best laid plans. For example, we had a case in which an Iraq War veteran blamed himself for failing to prevent a suicide bomb attack by recognizing the attacker as such and apprehending him. The *intention* of the attacker was to appear as anything other than a suicide bomber; thus, it would have been nearly impossible for our client to determine that the individual was a bomber given the information he had at the time. In another case, the work was to contextualize the enemy's intentions. This client could not make sense of why insurgents would be attacking when the forces were there to "liberate them." The veteran identified the thought, "They shouldn't have attacked us because we were there to help them." Through the process of Socratic dialogue regarding the Iraqi insurgents' likely intentions, the veteran and his wife began to appreciate the contextual factors for the insurgents' behaviors, namely that they did not perceive the military personnel as liberators but rather as occupiers. The veteran further concluded that the Iraqi insurgents probably believed at the time that surprise mortar attacks and other combat-related violence were the only means they had at their disposal to eject a foreign occupying force from their country and ensure their survival as a people.

The scenarios represent some of the more clear-cut cases of inappropriate blame. Nevertheless, it is very easy to fall prey to victim blame with the client and partner. As individuals embedded in our culture, we as clinicians are also inculcated with cultural messages about the justness of the world. We also want to maintain our beliefs that we can predict and control bad things from happening in spite of evidence to the contrary. This can lead us to inadvertently blame the victim as well, without careful thought about the intentions and circumstances surrounding the traumatic event.

In some cases, the intention *was* to do harm. That intentionality rests on a continuum that has to be evaluated in order to process the trauma context fully. Our legal system appreciates the dimensionality of intentionality in assigning different types of crimes (i.e., misdemeanors and felonies) and degrees of physical assault and murder (first degree, second degree, manslaughter). Those degrees are often designated based on the "clarity" of the person's intention at the time. The purpose of this discussion is to illustrate that even one's intentionality rests on a continuum and that there are a range of factors that must be evaluated before ascribing blame.

The important principle is for you to make the couple's thinking about the traumatic situation more complex or "big picture" by taking into account these important contextual variables about intentionality and state of mind and to encourage fair-minded and balanced thinking about the situation.

## *Situational Context*

In addition to appreciating fully the state of mind of those involved in a traumatic event by evaluating intentionality, it is also crucial that the couple take into account the situational context that was impinging on the individuals involved in the traumatic event. As discussed in the prior session, an important way in which traumatized individuals and couples can get stuck in their recovery is to neglect the situational factors at play that help determine a person's behavior in a given circumstance.

Important situational variables that must be taken into account include the actual environment (i.e., hot, cold, crowded), other events that transpired proximal to the event (e.g., interpersonal loss), personal and professional relationships (e.g., acquaintance, family), and consequences for alternative actions. For example, a service member who was in the field for days, just lost his best friend in a firefight the prior morning, and would be ridiculed by others if he did not engage in some act of overkilling needs to take all of that situational information into account when processing the context of his behavior and the traumatic event (see the following discussion for more information about acts of aggression committed by a PTSD+ partner during traumatic events). Another example might be a rape victim who blames herself for not reporting her crime. Was the perpetrator in her social circle? What consequences did she anticipate if she reported? Is there an assumption that there would have been positive outcomes if she had reported? A grueling trial might be a very negative consequence if she had chosen to report. Another example might be blaming an authority figure for her inaction. Were there potential untoward consequences if she would have acted? Does the traumatized person have all of the information that the authority figure had at the time in making her decision? One cannot know an outcome not chosen.

*It is important to remember that these two dimensions (intention and context) must be evaluated as they existed **at the time of the traumatic event(s)** and not as the person or significant other evaluates it with the benefit of time and distance.*

## Traumas Involving the Client's Aggression against Another

One important consideration when treating combat-related trauma is that deliberate aggression against another can be a job requirement. Other examples of employment in which aggression against another can occur in the line of duty and is sometimes sanctioned include police and security positions. Irrespective of whether a person's occupation includes aggressing against another at some point in time, the traumatized person's state of mind at the time is still relevant to putting the situation back into its proper context. The traumatized person may have been deliberate about aggressing against another person and, therefore, had the *proper* intentionality at the time of combat. In conceptualizing clients' stuck points and using that to guide the Socratic dialogue between the partners, the issues to consider are often more about the dimension of carefulness. To what degree did clients have the intention to follow the rules and regulations as best as they could, given the specific situation in which they found themselves? If their intention was to be as careful as they could in the very difficult circumstances found in modern warfare and a bad outcome occurred, they should not be blamed for their actions. If clients report that they were not as careful as they *should* have been, the therapist and their partner's work is to flesh out the circumstances that led to them not being as careful as they believe they should have been. Short of the intention to be careless, full blame is not appropriate. There are always situational demands impinging on clients at the time of the event that led to their behavior (e.g., exhaustion, mechanical failures, no specific guidance on what is the "right" thing to do). In other words, clients' *situational neglect* should be targeted. Clients and their partner may *wish* that the circumstances were not as they were but that does not necessarily mean that they did something for which they should be blamed. Self- or other-blame is appropriate if there is willful disregard of the rules and no extenuating circumstances.

Often, the work to be done to get clients unstuck when an index event involved their aggression against another revolves around characterological attributions or difficulty with accepting that they could do something that is inconsistent with how they want to construe themselves. With this type of stuck point, the idea is to challenge the notion that behavior in one situation generalizes to behavior in all situations. For example, was the client aggressive against others across all situations while he was in the military? Has he been aggressive, in general, since? Watch for strong, morally laden words that the couple might use and gently correct the use of this language to be more precise in labeling the situational context of the behavior. An example involves a client who was stuck on the characterological attribution that he was a "murderer" because during combat he had killed civilians who appeared to be enemy combatants. His wife did an excellent job of initiating Socratic dialogue with him to point out that he killed in the context of warfare and that he would have been a bad warrior if he hadn't. With the clinician's help, they also agreed that the term "murder" involves certain intentionality and circumstances and that his behavior did not fulfill these requirements.

A related and important note is that clinicians and clients alike tend to misuse the terms "atrocity" and "war crimes" in their descriptions and discussions. Bear in mind that the term "atrocity," like the term "insanity," has legal definitions and consequences and, therefore, is imbued with much judgment and negative affect. Sometimes the term applies, but it should be used judiciously and appropriately. Language is extremely important to construal of self and others in events, and misuse of these terms can have negative consequences for the well-being of the traumatized person and the partner.

The second type of stuck point relates to the client and the partner developing a more multidimensional and textured view of self and others. Social psychological research indicates that most of us would aggress against another in certain circumstances (e.g., Haney et al., 1973; Milgram, 1974). The work to untangle the stuck point is to appreciate fully the extenuating circumstances that were at play in the situation and to accept fully that one is capable of acting or not acting, given those circumstances. The client may wish that he or she or someone else acted differently, but they didn't. What does that mean about him or her or the others? It means that we are all human and neglect the powerful circumstances that are sometimes overdetermining. It doesn't necessarily mean that we are to blame for an event occurring in the first place. If the client did something that is indeed out of the bounds of the situation, then the work is to accept that good people sometimes do bad things, but their role in the events doesn't necessarily make them bad people.

## *Forgiveness*

There is definitely a role for forgiveness or repentance in this therapy in order to bring closure to traumatic events. However, there is an important caution about forgiveness: Inappropriately placed forgiveness of self or others can also inhibit processing of traumatic events and cause stuckness. In our experience, forgiveness does not fully work if the client is trying to forgive him- or herself or another for unintentional outcomes or negative outcomes that resulted in spite of careful behavior. Sometimes a client will rush to forgiveness of self or other in an attempt to avoid the traumatic memory. A client will foreclose on processing by seeking to forgive in order not to approach the traumatic memory. Also, forgiveness implies blame, and if inappropriate or misplaced blame is ascribed, then forgiveness is unlikely to work as a means of decreasing PTSD symptoms. The symptoms, and especially intrusions, will continue until there is more realistic or reasonable allocation of blame. Thus, forgiveness should be reserved until after a careful review of the mental states of those involved and a full appreciation of the situational context in which the event(s) occurred.

Give the couple *Getting U.N.S.T.U.C.K. Regarding Blame* (*Handout 9.1*) and begin reviewing the key concepts to convey to the couple. Your goal with regard to blame, like with other trauma-relevant themes, is to help the couple develop a more textured, multifaceted, and complex way of thinking about the concept. In addition, you want to make sure that if there is blame that needs to be placed, depending on intentionality/state of mind and situational variables, upon whom should it be placed and how much? There *may* be blame to place on the person with

PTSD or others involved in the traumatic experience(s). However, instruct the couple that we first want to make sure that the blame is being appropriately placed, because inappropriately placed blame can be a barrier to successful recovery.

Begin walking the couple through the specific cognitive barriers listed on *Getting U.N.S.T.U.C.K. Regarding Blame* (Handout 9.1) as it pertains to looking back on traumatic events. Note that some of the barriers related to acceptance from the prior session apply to blame, which reinforces and expands upon these important concepts with the couple.

*I am going to transition us now to talk about blame for the traumatic event(s). There is a natural tendency to want to place blame on someone for bad things happening. It is one of the ways in which we try to exert control and believe that we can prevent future bad things from happening. However, as we discussed in our last session, bad things can just happen, without anyone intending for them to happen. Sometimes the best laid plans do not lead to good outcomes. Ill-placed blame can keep you stuck and impede your recovery from PTSD.*

*In this session we are going to focus on two things:*

1. *Is there "blame" to be placed on someone?*
2. *If so, how much?*

*In this therapy, we use the term "blame" in a very specific way. Blame involves intending to do harm to someone or something and/or reckless behavior that results in bad outcomes. It is important for us to think about what happened in terms of whether you or someone else purposefully intended to do something that caused harm.*

*One way of thinking about degrees of blame is to think about how crimes are categorized in our legal system. All behaviors are not seen as equal in the eyes of the law. Depending on a person's intentions and behavior, he or she may or may not even get charged for causing harm to another. Depending on intentions **at the time** and the degree of carelessness, he or she might get charged with different levels of crimes (misdemeanors vs. felony; degrees of murder or assault).*

*In addition, some of those ways of thinking that we discussed last week related to acceptance of the traumatic event are also relevant to blame. For example, **just-world thinking** can be at play. If something bad happened to you, and you believe bad things happen to bad people, you may blame yourself for the bad thing happening. With **hindsight** bias you might be looking back on the situation with the information that you have now after the fact to believe that you or someone else **should** have known and, therefore, done something different, and that something different would have led to a positive outcome. We discussed the "happily-ever-after" or "fairytale" thinking that you can fall prey to as a result of hindsight bias.*

*Finally, you'll remember that we discussed our human tendency to disregard important information about the situation that influences our behavior: **situational neglect**. You or someone else might have done something that you consider against your moral code or contrary to how you want to see yourself. To see the big picture, we have to remember all of the situation and not just the tunnel vision.*

## In-Session Practice:
## U.N.S.T.U.C.K. Regarding Blame and Other Stuck Points

After this portion of the psychoeducation is complete, refer back to the couple's responses on the TIQ-I (*Handout 1.5*) pertaining to the question about why the traumatic event occurred. Determine whether there is any inappropriately placed blame on self or others. Urge the couple to consider forgiveness, if necessary, only after appropriately considering the whole situation and, specifically, intentionality and situational variables. Have the couple turn their chairs to face each other to use the U.N.S.T.U.C.K. process to begin to address stuck points related to blame. In determining the stuck points to work on in this area, it is helpful to listen closely to the PTSD+ partner's reactions to the psychoeducation regarding blame. When he or she hears the notions about intentionality and situational context, and as you solicit examples, the PTSD+ partner will often make comments about the specific barriers in his or her own rendition of events. Other suggested questions to make sure that you elicit stuck points related to blame include:

- Are there parts that you blame yourself for?
- Are there parts that you blame others for?
- Did you (or someone else) intend for _____ to happen?
- Do you think that you (or someone else) did something wrong to cause _____ to happen?
- What do you think you should have done or not have done to prevent _____?
- Did you or anyone else have any other choices given the situation?

Like in previous sessions, ask a partner to write the stuck point in the circle of *The Big Picture* worksheet (*Handout 9.2*) and coach the couple in their use of the U.N.S.T.U.C.K. process. It is important that you do as much as possible to turn the work over to the couple. In this final phase of therapy, you want the couple to have as much experience as possible using the U.N.S.T.U.C.K. process on their own. We often "plant" questions for the partner to ask to facilitate the Socratic dialogue between the couple, such as:

- "Pete, what are you curious about with Susan regarding her belief that she should have done _____?"
- "Ann, what question do you have for Tom about what his commanding officer was thinking at the time of the ambush?"
- "John, are there questions that you have for Pat about what he thinks he did wrong in the situation?"

After completing the U.N.S.T.U.C.K. process, consider with the couple whether there is any problem solving/decision making that they should embark upon. The problem solving can be as simple as "How can we carry out the "K = Keep practicing" part of the U.N.S.T.U.C.K. process?"

While listening to the couple using the U.N.S.T.U.C.K. process, monitor for other stuck points that emerge during this session to be put on the *Stuck Point List* (*Handout 8.1*). The more stuck points that can be identified in session with the couple and placed on the list, the greater the chance that they can be effectively addressed out of session.

Following is an excerpt from a session focused on blame involving an Iraq War veteran who found the dead and mutilated body of a young Iraqi boy killed by insurgents because his father had cooperated with American soldiers. One of the client's stuck points involved the belief that there are universally held rules of combat that should govern people's actions, even in war (this case was originally presented in Fredman, Monson, & Adair, 2011).

THERAPIST: Let's try something out with this U.N.S.T.U.C.K. process. It sounds like what you're saying is that they shouldn't have done this because that violated these rules of humanity that you had going into Iraq: that there are rules of humanity—that, even in a war, there are certain things that you don't do, even if you're trying to win. I'm going to ask the two of you to evaluate this thought together. Although I'm going to be asking some questions, I would like you, Sue, to, as you can, chime in with curious thoughts as we start putting the idea that they shouldn't have done this on the table (N—Notice your thought). We could also turn the thought on its head and say, "Why shouldn't they have done this?" I'd like you to take a unified and curious approach (U) to the thought that the insurgents shouldn't have tortured and killed this child . . . I know that this might seem kind of crazy or radical but—what are some alternatives to "They shouldn't have done this?" that you guys have come up with (S—(Brain)Storming alternatives)?

MARTIN: It's not that they shouldn't have done it. It's "How could they do it?" It's that . . .

THERAPIST: It sounds like underneath there's the idea that they shouldn't have tortured and killed an innocent child.

MARTIN: Yeah, I mean, definitely no. Yeah, I just remember, after it happened, I just couldn't comprehend how they could do it. I don't know.

THERAPIST: So the work is to get you to be able to comprehend that. Not to say it's okay to kill and torture children, but to be able to comprehend how they could do that, because truly I think that's what's keeping you stuck . . . You said, "I can't make sense of it," and I think that's what's driving the PTSD and the anger and the irritability.

SUE: Is there the possibility that they did it to protect their people, kind of the same way you were trying to protect your people by trying to get information from the father?

MARTIN: Yeah, it could be. Definitely.

THERAPIST: That's a great question. Could you ask more about that?

SUE: Sure. I guess, do you think that they were . . .

MARTIN: Yeah, try to look at it from their point of view.

SUE: Right.

MARTIN: Yeah, definitely. Yeah . . . I don't know. All right, I'm sorry, killing people is all right, well, it's not all right, but there are humane ways to do things . . . They were doing it to create a bigger impact than just torturing this kid. They were trying to run the neighborhood.

SUE: Right, but in their minds, what they were doing was probably right.

MARTIN: Yeah, it was. Definitely, it was.

SUE: They probably thought that if the Army, or whoever was getting information . . . it would affect their life, their lifestyle, and they probably thought a child's life versus a whole community's life or whole area's life is worth showing this man that there are consequences for cooperating with the Americans. They thought it might stand out to the community and send a message. And ultimately this message would help to keep them safer.

THERAPIST: Martin, before you respond, could you paraphrase what Sue said?

MARTIN: That they had the same intentions as we do—to protect the people in the neighborhood—but they just have a different way of doing it. Is that it?

SUE: Right, and they have different views as to what's humane and not because of their circumstances. You had said before it's kind of almost like survival of the fittest over there, everyone kind of feeds off everyone else. It's one of those things where it's "kill or be killed" sometimes in some situations.

THERAPIST: It sounds like what you're saying is that to protect themselves they made an example of this child. What do you think of that, Martin? (T—Testing alternatives)

MARTIN: Yeah, I guess the more extreme you do something, the more people see it or fear it, or whatever it is, and obviously torturing and killing a little kid, that's pretty . . . crazy.

THERAPIST: So, Sue, could you start writing stuff down as we're talking about this? You asked a really good question, so I want to make sure we get that down and then get this other stuff down too.

SUE: Sure, so what was my question?

MARTIN: The aspect of the people who did it, that their intentions were the same as ours. (Testing alternatives)

THERAPIST: To protect their community. It was really great that you came up with that.

SUE: What happened at Abu Ghraib prison—it is kind of the same thing.

MARTIN: Yeah, but I don't think it was to the same degree.

THERAPIST: Are you saying that Abu Ghraib was sort of an example on a continuum?

MARTIN: Good point. I think it could eventually get to the same extent.

## Shrinking PTSD through Approach

From the *Avoidance List* (*Handout 3.2*), determine the next person, place, situation, or feeling that will be approached prior to the next session. Record the item on the *OOSA summary* (*Handout 9.3*) and ask the couple to write about how it went.

As in previous sessions, anticipate with the couple barriers to the success of carrying out the approach behavior and preemptively problem solve how those behaviors might be overcome. Refer them to the PROUD acronym in *Handout 4.3* to help strategize maximizing the benefits of the approach exercise.

## Out-of-Session Assignments

Orient the couple to the *OOSA summary* (*Handout 9.3*) for this session and point out the following assignments:

- Together, read *Getting U.N.S.T.U.C.K. Regarding Blame* (*Handout 9.1*).
- Have the couple use the U.N.S.T.U.C.K. process with *The Big Picture* (*Handout 9.2*) at least four times prior to the next session (more if they are willing). The PTSD+ partner should nominate at least one trauma-related cognition and the other partner should nominate any cognitions that he or she is struggling with (trauma related or not). Prioritize partners' stuck points that may impede their own (in dual-PTSD cases) or their partner's recovery (e.g., "My partner being distressed means her PTSD is worse"). Each partner should also nominate a relationship-related cognition that each has.

    During the session, pay attention to thoughts expressed by each member of the couple that would be helpful for them to work on outside of session. This will help increase adherence and help you to be more targeted in your work with them to resolve PTSD and other mental health symptoms and to improve their relationship. We recommend that the therapist help the couple to generate and record on individual *Big Picture* (*Handout 9.2*) worksheets the specific thoughts that they will work on together outside of the session as well as any identified stuck points on their *Stuck Point List* (*Handout 8.1*).
- Ask the couple to spend 5 minutes each day using their best communication skills with one another (*Handout 9.3*).
- Remind the couple of the item chosen from the *Avoidance List* (*Handout 3.2*) to be approached prior to the next session and ask them to record how it went.

## Check-Out

Ask the couple how the session was for each of them. Are there any lingering concerns or questions? What do they want to take with them from the session to improve their relationship and PTSD? Infuse hopefulness and predict success in completing the OOSAs as they leave the session.

HANDOUT 9.1

# Getting U.N.S.T.U.C.K. Regarding Blame

One of the barriers to successful recovery from PTSD can be misplaced or extreme blame. The key to getting unstuck is to stop avoiding the memory of the event and to appreciate fully the **entire** picture or context of the situation. There may or may not be someone to *blame* for a bad outcome. There is a tendency to want to blame oneself or others for bad things happening in an effort to regain a sense of control over the situation.

## HOW DO WE ASSESS BLAME FOR AN EVENT?

There are two factors to consider when determining whether there is blame for an event and if so, how much.

- *Intentions/state of mind.* What were your or others' intentions at the time of the event? In other words, did you *mean* for the bad outcome to occur? Did others intend for the bad outcome to occur?
- *Situation at the time.* What was going on at the time that might have impacted your or others' behavior?

**There are several types of tunnel vision that can get one stuck regarding blame, including:**

- *Just-world thinking.* "Good things happen to good people. Bad things happen to bad people." If a bad thing happened to you, you might assume that you did something bad or are to blame for the traumatic event happening to you. Also, if a bad thing happened and you were involved, you might assume that you or someone else did a bad thing or are bad people.
- *Hindsight bias.* "I or someone else should have known." You might also think that you or someone else should have done something different and presume that this alternative action would have led to a positive versus negative outcome (i.e., *fairytale thinking*). Sometimes the best laid plans at the time don't lead to the best outcomes.
- *Situational neglect.* If you did something that you consider against your moral code or contrary to how you want to see yourself or others do see you, remember that we have a tendency to overlook the powerful situational factors that influence our choices and our behaviors. Good people do bad things, too, in certain circumstances.

It is incredibly important to put things back in perspective, given a view of the big picture when assessing blame of yourself and others. Once the entire picture regarding blame is developed, then you can work on forgiving yourself or others **if that is appropriate**. Your first job as a couple is to figure out if there is blame to be placed and if so, whom and how much that person is to be blamed.

Forgiving yourself or others is appropriate to bring closure to traumatic events. However, if you attempt to forgive before you have done a good job of figuring out if there is blame deserving forgiveness, then forgiveness is unlikely to work.

---

From *Cognitive-Behavioral Conjoint Therapy for PTSD: Harnessing the Healing Power of Relationships* by Candice M. Monson and Steffany J. Fredman. Copyright 2012 by The Guilford Press. Permission to photocopy this handout is granted to purchasers of this book for personal use only (see copyright page for details).

HANDOUT 9.2

# The Big Picture

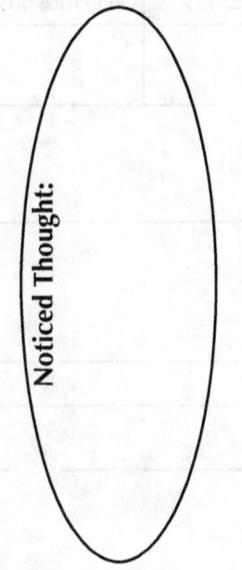

Noticed Thought:

C: *Feelings?*

K:

*Behaviors?*

U = United and curious
N = Notice your thought
S = (Brain)Storm alternatives
T = Test them out
U = Use the most balanced
C = Changed feelings and behaviors
K = Keep practicing

From *Cognitive-Behavioral Conjoint Therapy for PTSD: Harnessing the Healing Power of Relationships* by Candice M. Monson and Steffany J. Fredman. Copyright 2012 by The Guilford Press. Permission to photocopy this handout is granted to purchasers of this book for personal use only (see copyright page for details).

177

HANDOUT 9.3

# Out-of-Session Assignments
## Session 9. Getting U.N.S.T.U.C.K. Regarding Blame

1. Together, read *Getting U.N.S.T.U.C.K. Regarding Blame* (Handout 9.1).

2. Use the U.N.S.T.U.C.K. process together at least four times prior to the next session. You should each work on two thoughts, one individually oriented and one relationship related, that can be drawn from the *Stuck Point List* (Handout 8.1). At least one of the individually oriented thoughts should be trauma related. Try on the new thoughts and notice what emotions and behaviors follow from these thoughts. Use your problem-solving/decision-making skills to figure out how you as a couple will use these new behaviors.

3. Spend 5 minutes each day using your best communication skills with one another. Place a checkmark below for each day you practiced.

| Sunday | Monday | Tuesday | Wednesday | Thursday | Friday | Saturday |
|--------|--------|---------|-----------|----------|--------|----------|
|        |        |         |           |          |        |          |

4. Shrinking PTSD through Approach:

_____
(people, place, situation, feeling)

Write about how it went:

_____
_____

**Next appointment:** _____ @ _____

---

From *Cognitive-Behavioral Conjoint Therapy for PTSD: Harnessing the Healing Power of Relationships* by Candice M. Monson and Steffany J. Fredman. Copyright 2012 by The Guilford Press. Permission to photocopy this handout is granted to purchasers of this book for personal use only (see copyright page for details).

# SESSION 10

# Trust

---

**SUMMARY OF SESSION CONTENT**

### Goals

- Reinforce the couple's work with the U.N.S.T.U.C.K. process, and troubleshoot any difficulties they are having.
- Address problematic core here-and-now beliefs related to trust that may be maintaining PTSD and relationship discord.
- Highlight that there are different types of trust and that these types of trust exist on continua.

### Key Interventions

1. Review of Out-of-Session Assignments
   - *Getting U.N.S.T.U.C.K. Regarding Blame* (Handout 9.1)
   - *The Big Picture* (Handout 9.2)
   - *Communication Skills Practice* (Handout 9.3)
   - *Shrinking PTSD through Approach* (Handout 9.3)
2. Introduction to Trust (*Getting U.N.S.T.U.C.K. Regarding Trust*, Handout 10.1)
   - Convey that traumatic events impact trust by confirming previously held negative beliefs or disrupting previously held positive beliefs.
   - Discuss the three principles regarding trust (i.e., applies to self and others, is a multidimensional construct, and healthy thoughts are balanced ones).
3. In-Session Practice: U.N.S.T.U.C.K. Regarding Trust and Other Stuck Points
   - Refer to the couple's TIQ-I (*Handout 1.5*) regarding trust barriers.
   - Help the couple generate any stuck points related to trust.
   - Use problem solving/decision making after U.N.S.T.U.C.K.
4. Shrinking PTSD through Approach
   - Determine at least one person, place, situation, or feeling to be approached.
   - Record the item on the *OOSA summary* (Handout 10.3).
5. Out-of-Session Assignments (Handout 10.3)
   - *Getting U.N.S.T.U.C.K. Regarding Trust* (Handout 10.1)
   - *The Big Picture* (Handout 10.2)
   - *Communication Skills Practice* (Handout 10.3)
   - *Shrinking PTSD through Approach* (Handout 10.3)
6. Check-Out

*Administer the patient and partner versions of PCL/relationship happiness.

## Review of Out-of-Session Assignments

• *Getting U.N.S.T.U.C.K. Regarding Blame* (Handout 9.1). Inquire whether either member of the couple had any questions about this handout.

• *The Big Picture* (Handout 9.2). Have the couple explain their use of the U.N.S.T.U.C.K. process on their respective cognitions. Reinforce the couple's hard work in doing the assignment, troubleshoot what got in the way of completing the assignment, and/or coach the couple on ways in which the U.N.S.T.U.C.K. procedure and use of *The Big Picture* could be optimized.

• *Communication Skills Practice* (Handout 9.3). Inquire about the couple's use of good communication skills since the last session.

• *Shrinking PTSD through Approach* (Handout 9.3). Review how the *in vivo* assignment went and reinforce any approach behavior and couple-level facilitation of such. Troubleshoot ways in which the couple may have accommodated avoidance. If the couple was successful in approaching an item off of the *Avoidance List* (Handout 3.2), in some way note this on their list (e.g., cross it out if no longer avoided, place a checkmark if previously assigned but still working on it).

## Introduction to Trust

We offer a reminder that this and next three sessions are related to core belief areas (i.e., trust, power/control, emotional closeness, physical closeness) that are usually disrupted by traumatic events in those with PTSD if there were previous positive beliefs in these areas or can seem to be reinforced if previous negative beliefs were held in these areas (McCann & Pearlman, 1990). It is helpful to think of them as **conclusions that traumatized individuals take away from the traumatic event.** In this way, they are "downstream" consequences of appraisals of the traumatic event. Therefore, when prioritizing stuck points for the couple to work on, it is important to remember that accurate appraisal of the traumatic event(s) usually change here-and-now thoughts in these areas. **Thus, a more accurate picture of the past can have important ramifications for the present.**

The prior two sessions were explicitly focused on correcting appraisals about the traumatic event(s). **This session and the three that follow should prioritize reappraisal of the traumatic event(s)** *to the extent that there are remaining appraisals that have not been examined or adequately addressed.* Psychoeducation about the topics of these sessions (trust, power/control, emotional closeness, physical closeness) should still be presented but used as a jumping-off point to determine how the couple's trauma appraisals disrupted or confirmed beliefs in the given topic area.

With this important case conceptualization point in mind, transition out of the review of OOSAs to provide psychoeducation about **trust** as it relates to self and others. It is important to convey that traumatic events often impact trust, whether they confirm previously held negative beliefs or disrupt previously held positive beliefs.

In providing psychoeducation about trust of self and others, the most important principles to convey are that **(1) trust applies to self and others, (2) it is a multidimensional construct, and (3) healthy thoughts about trust are balanced ones.** Orient the couple to *Getting U.N.S.T.U.C.K. Regarding Trust* (Handout 10.1).

*I'd like to draw your attention to this handout about our next topic: trust. When someone is traumatized, trust of oneself and/or others can be shaken. You'll notice that there are two columns on this handout: one focused on beliefs about self-trust and one about trust of each other and other people. Self-trust is the belief that you can rely upon your own perceptions or judgments, and trust of others is the belief that the promises and actions of your partner or others can be relied upon. If you had a history of not trusting yourself prior to the traumatic event, the traumatic event might seem to reinforce that you can't trust yourself. If you trusted yourself pretty well prior to the trauma(s), the trauma(s) might shake your trust of yourself. The same applies to your trust of your partner and others. Depending on your beliefs prior to the traumatic event, the trauma can either seem to confirm or shake your beliefs in this area.*

*There are several important parts to Getting U.N.S.T.U.C.K. Regarding Trust. All of them are about having balanced, big-picture thoughts. First, there are many types of things about which you trust yourself and others—for example, trust about someone being on time or choosing good friends. The second important part of getting U.N.S.T.U.C.K. is to remember that trust exists on a continuum, meaning that there are shades of gray about how much you trust yourself or others. People with PTSD tend to think of trust as an either/or, like a light switch. We'll be working together to put a "dimmer" on that switch to consider different levels of trust. On the sheet it shows us that trust is on a spectrum and is dependent on the type of trust [refer to Handout 10.1].*

In addition to psychoeducation about balanced thoughts regarding trust, it is also important to convey to the couple how to approach trust of oneself and others when evidence does not yet exist and what to do when the inevitable concerns about trust arise. The principles here are to **adopt a nonjudgmental stance initially, until there is evidence upon which to form an opinion.** It is important to convey that one's opinion can and should change based on new information. Eliciting an example from the couple of an instance in which an opinion about someone changed from the negative to the positive based on new information is helpful to the psychoeducation but also to combating the negative attentional filter that accompanies PTSD.

Stress to the couple that, in the life of their relationship, they are likely to have occasions in which their trust of one another or of themselves will be questioned. Normalize this as part of the natural course of human relationships.

*If someone seems to have made a mistake, take the time to test out the interpretation. In other words, collect information before coming to any conclusion. If mistakes were made, then notice how you, your partner, or others respond to those mistakes. Actions to repair and times in which the person is trustworthy should gradually increase trust. Inaction and/or continued untrustworthy behavior should further decrease trust. The caution is against going to extremes in either direction.*

*Let's talk about situations in which you don't have good information about your ability to trust yourself, your partner, or others. Is your inclination to distrust until proven otherwise? Guilty until proven innocent? Are there any downsides to that approach? Our recommendation is to make no judgments until you have good information, or at least recognize when you do make snap judgments. Ideally, you assume a neutral stance and adjust your opinions as information comes in.*

*In human relationships, it is inevitable to worry about being betrayed or to experience actual breaches of trust. What if you suspect a betrayal of your own or others' trust? Do you check it out first, or do you assume the worst? Assume the best?*

*Our prescription is to be open-minded before coming to any conclusions and check out your thoughts using the U.N.S.TU.C.K. process before concluding that a betrayal has occurred.*

*If a mistake has been made that affects your **level** [stress added here to punctuate its occurring on a continuum] of trust of yourself, your partner, or others, take time to notice how that mistake is handled. Are there attempts to repair? Are you or others acting trustworthy over time? Use this information to adjust your level of trust, fighting the temptation to immediately cut ties, lose all trust, and/or conclude that a single event defines your or others' characters. What do think was behind your partner's actions? Sometimes it is something benign or totally unrelated to what you assumed your partner was thinking.*

## In-Session Practice:
## U.N.S.T.U.C.K. Regarding Trust and Other Stuck Points

After the psychoeducation is complete, review with the couple their responses to the TIQ-I (*Handout 1.5*) as a starting point for identifying stuck points regarding trust. This is also an opportunity to monitor progress in thoughts over the course of the therapy. The goal is to spend only a few minutes reviewing the TIQ-I so that they can identify their stuck points and begin their in-session U.N.S.T.U.C.K. process. The focus should be toward getting the couple to discuss these issues together, with you serving as a role model for Socratic dialogue.

*Let's look at what the two of you wrote at the beginning of therapy about your trust beliefs. You have both done a lot of work since you first wrote these statements and so the thoughts you have now about trust may already be different from the ones you wrote down weeks ago, but that's okay. We can note the changes, and reviewing your original responses will jump-start our discussion.*

After the couple shares their responses to the TIQ-I, have them turn their chairs to face each other to use the U.N.S.T.U.C.K. process to begin to address stuck points related to trust and any other stuck points that have been prioritized to be addressed.

As in previous sessions, ask a partner to write the stuck point in the circle of *The Big Picture* (*Handout 10.2*) and coach the couple in their use of the U.N.S.T.U.C.K. process. It is important that you continue to strive to turn the work over to the couple so that they have as much experience as possible using the U.N.S.T.U.C.K. process on their own. Continue to "plant" questions for the partner to ask to facilitate the Socratic dialogue between the couple.

Examples of balanced beliefs regarding trust that you might coach the couple toward include:

- "I can trust *some* authority figures in *many* circumstances."
- "I can trust myself in most all areas."
- "I can trust my partner on the important stuff, but not to be on time."

**The emphasis is on nonabsolute and balanced language.**

After completing a worksheet, it is important to translate balanced thoughts into action. Consider with the couple whether there is any problem solving/decision making that they should embark upon. The problem solving can be as simple as "How can we carry out the 'K = Keep practicing' part of the U.N.S.T.U.C.K. process?"

While listening to the couple using the U.N.S.T.U.C.K. process, monitor for other stuck points that emerge during this session to be put on the *Stuck Point List* (*Handout 8.1*). The more stuck points that can be identified in session with the couple and placed on the list, the greater the chance that they can be effectively addressed out of session.

## Shrinking PTSD through Approach

From the *Avoidance List* (*Handout 3.2*), determine the person, place, situation, or feeling that will be approached prior to the next session. Record the item on the *OOSA summary* (*Handout 10.3*) and ask the couple to write about how it went.

As in previous sessions, anticipate with the couple barriers to the success of carrying out the approach behavior and preemptively problem solve how those behaviors might be overcome. Refer them to the PROUD acronym in *Handout 4.3* to help strategize maximizing the benefits of the approach exercise.

## Out-of-Session Assignments

Orient the couple to the *OOSA summary* (*Handout 10.3*) for this session and point out the following assignments:

- Together, read *Getting U.N.S.T.U.C.K. Regarding Trust* (*Handout 10.1*).
- Have the couple use the U.N.S.T.U.C.K. process with *The Big Picture* (*Handout 10.2*) at least four times prior to the next session (more if they are willing). The PTSD+ partner should nominate at least one trauma-related cognition and the other partner should nominate any cognitions that he or she is struggling with (trauma related or not). Prioritize partners' stuck points that may impede their own (in dual-PTSD cases) or their partner's recovery (e.g., "My partner being distressed means her PTSD is worse"). Each partner should also nominate a relationship-related cognition that each has.

    During the session, pay attention to thoughts expressed by each member of the couple that would be helpful for them to work on outside of session. This will help increase adherence and help you to be more targeted in your work with them to resolve PTSD and other mental health symptoms and to improve their relationship. We recommend

that you help the couple to generate and record on individual *Big Picture* (*Handout 10.2*) worksheets the specific thoughts that they will work on together outside of the session as well as any identified stuck points on their *Stuck Point List* (*Handout 8.1*).
- Ask the couple to spend 5 minutes each day using their best communication skills with one another (*Handout 10.3*).
- Remind the couple of the item chosen from the *Avoidance List* (*Handout 3.2*) to be approached prior to the next session and ask them to record how it went.

## Check-Out

Ask the couple how the session was for each of them. Are there any lingering concerns or questions? What do they want to take with them from the session to improve their relationship and PTSD? Infuse hopefulness and predict success in completing the OOSAs as they leave the session.

HANDOUT 10.1

# Getting U.N.S.T.U.C.K. Regarding Trust

**Beliefs Related to Self.** The belief that one can rely upon one's own perceptions or judgments. This belief is an important part of our self-esteem and serves to protect us from harm.

*The traumatic event(s) may have made you question your ability to trust your perceptions of situations or judgments about people and circumstances. You may have concluded from the event that you can't trust yourself to make decisions or act positively in situations.*

- Do I believe that I generally have good judgment about people and situations?
- Can I trust how I will behave in different situations?
- Do I "read" situations well?

**Beliefs Related to Partner and Others.** The belief that the promises and actions of your partner and others can be relied upon.

*Traumatic events often include other people who you believe caused you harm. Thus, you may have come to believe that others cannot be trusted to have your best interests at heart. If people around you after the event were blaming, distant, or unsupportive, your belief in their trustworthiness may also have been challenged.*

- Do I think that anyone can be truly trusted?
- Do I assume that others will inevitably hurt or betray me?
- Can I trust my partner to be there for me?

**There are many different types of trust**—for example, trusting your partner to be on time, trusting yourself to choose good friends, trusting someone to pay you back, trusting someone to keep a secret, trusting you or your partner's money management skills.

**Trust is on a continuum.** When people have been traumatized, they often think of trust as an "on/off" switch: "I trust myself or I don't. I trust my partner completely or not at all." Healthy trust is on a continuum (or has shades of gray) and is dependent on the category of trust above—for example, trust in my partner to:

Pay the bills    ----------------------------↑----------------------------

Keep a secret    ------------------------------------------------------↑

Be on time       ----------------------------------------------------------
                 ↑
                 Not at all                                      Completely

### RESOLUTION: BALANCE

When evaluating trust in yourself, your partner, or others, it is helpful to make no judgments until you have good information—not innocent or guilty until proven so. On the basis of this information, you can change your levels of trust.

*(cont.)*

---

From *Cognitive-Behavioral Conjoint Therapy for PTSD: Harnessing the Healing Power of Relationships* by Candice M. Monson and Steffany J. Fredman. Copyright 2012 by The Guilford Press. Permission to photocopy this handout is granted to purchasers of this book for personal use only (see copyright page for details).

# Getting U.N.S.T.U.C.K. Regarding Trust *(page 2 of 2)*

Also, you, your partner, and others will make mistakes that can affect your trust. It is important to first test out whether a mistake has been made by seeking information. If a mistake has been made, it is **much** more important what you and others do with those mistakes. You will be tempted to go to extremes: "I can't trust myself" or "I can't trust him/her."

**Examples of more balanced, "big-picture" thinking are:**

- "I can trust my judgments in many, but not all, areas."
- "I can trust myself to make good decisions when it comes to _____, but might seek counsel when it comes to _____."
- "I trust that my partner will be dependable when it comes to all things except time management."
- "I can trust Tom to lend me money, but not to keep a secret from our friends."

# HANDOUT 10.2

## The Big Picture

U = United and curious
N = Notice your thought
S = (Brain)**S**torm alternatives
T = Test them out
U = Use the most balanced
C = Changed feelings and behaviors
K = Keep practicing

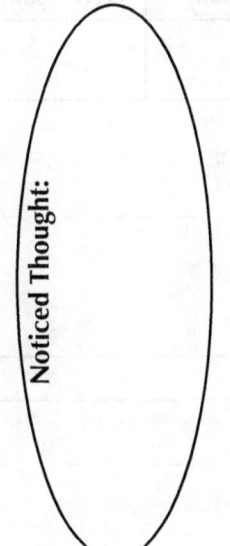

Noticed Thought:

C: *Feelings?*

*Behaviors?*

K:

From *Cognitive-Behavioral Conjoint Therapy for PTSD: Harnessing the Healing Power of Relationships* by Candice M. Monson and Steffany J. Fredman. Copyright 2012 by The Guilford Press. Permission to photocopy this handout is granted to purchasers of this book for personal use only (see copyright page for details).

HANDOUT 10.3

# Out-of-Session Assignments
## Session 10. Getting U.N.S.T.U.C.K. Regarding Trust

1. Together, read *Getting U.N.S.T.U.C.K. Regarding Trust* (Handout 10.1).

2. Use the U.N.S.T.U.C.K. process together at least four times prior to the next session. You should each work on two thoughts, one individually oriented and one relationship related, which can be drawn from the *Stuck Point List* (Handout 8.1). At least one of the individually oriented thoughts should be trauma related. Try on the new thoughts and notice what emotions and behaviors follow from these thoughts. Use your problem-solving/decision-making skills to figure out how you as a couple will use these new behaviors.

3. Spend 5 minutes each day using your best communication skills with one another. Place a checkmark below for each day you practiced.

| Sunday | Monday | Tuesday | Wednesday | Thursday | Friday | Saturday |
|--------|--------|---------|-----------|----------|--------|----------|
|        |        |         |           |          |        |          |

4. Shrinking PTSD through Approach:

_____

(people, place, situation, feeling)

Write about how it went:

_____

_____

**Next appointment:** _____ @ _____

---

From *Cognitive-Behavioral Conjoint Therapy for PTSD: Harnessing the Healing Power of Relationships* by Candice M. Monson and Steffany J. Fredman. Copyright 2012 by The Guilford Press. Permission to photocopy this handout is granted to purchasers of this book for personal use only (see copyright page for details).

# SESSION 11

# Control

---

### SUMMARY OF SESSION CONTENT

#### Goals

- Address overgeneralized here-and-now problematic core beliefs related to control that may be maintaining PTSD and relationship discord.
- Emphasize that there is variability in what people can and cannot control and that healthy relationships involve sharing control.

#### Key Interventions

1. Review of Out-of-Session Assignments
   - *Getting U.N.S.T.U.C.K. Regarding Trust* (Handout 10.1)
   - *The Big Picture* (Handout 10.2)
   - *Communication Skills Practice* (Handout 10.3)
   - *Shrinking PTSD through Approach* (Handout 10.3)
2. Introduction to Control (*Getting U.N.S.T.U.C.K. Regarding Control*, Handout 11.1)
   - Convey that traumatic events impact control by seemingly confirming previously held negative beliefs or disrupting previously held positive beliefs.
   - Discuss the principles regarding control of self and others (i.e., some things can be controlled, but not everything; healthy relationships involve sharing control).
3. In-Session Practice: U.N.S.T.U.C.K. Regarding Control and Other Stuck Points
   - Refer to the couple's TIQ-I (*Handout 1.5*) regarding control barriers.
   - Help the couple generate any stuck points related to control.
   - Use problem solving/decision making after U.N.S.T.U.C.K.
4. Shrinking PTSD through Approach
   - Determine at least one person, place, situation, or feeling to be approached.
   - Record the item on the *OOSA summary* (Handout 11.3).
5. Out-of-Session Assignments (*Handout 11.3*)
   - *Getting U.N.S.T.U.C.K. Regarding Control* (Handout 11.1)
   - *The Big Picture* (Handout 11.2)
   - *Communication Skills Practice* (Handout 11.3)
   - *Shrinking PTSD through Approach* (Handout 11.3)
6. Check-Out

---

\*Administer the patient and partner versions of PCL/relationship happiness.

## Review of Out-of-Session Assignments

- *Getting U.N.S.T.U.C.K. Regarding Trust (Handout 10.1)*. Inquire whether either member of the couple had any questions about this handout.

- *The Big Picture (Handout 10.2)*. Have the couple explain their use of the U.N.S.T.U.C.K. process on their respective cognitions. Reinforce the couple's hard work in doing the assignment, troubleshoot what got in the way of completing the assignment, and/or coach the couple on ways in which the U.N.S.T.U.C.K. procedure and use of *The Big Picture* could be optimized.

- *Communication Skills Practice (Handout 10.3)*. Inquire about the couple's use of good communication skills since the last session.

- *Shrinking PTSD through Approach (Handout 10.3)*. Review how the *in vivo* assignment went and reinforce any approach behavior and couple-level facilitation of such. Troubleshoot ways in which the couple may have accommodated avoidance. If the couple was successful in approaching an item off of the *Avoidance List (Handout 3.2)*, in some way note this on their list (e.g., cross it out if no longer avoided, place a checkmark if previously assigned but still working on it more).

## Introduction to Control

Transition out of the review of OOSAs to provide psychoeducation about **control** as it relates to self and others. Like issues of trust, traumatic events often affect control cognitions, whether they confirm previously held negative beliefs or disrupt previously held positive beliefs. It is important to remember that accurate appraisal of the traumatic event(s) usually changes here-and-now thoughts about control of oneself and others. Thus, a more accurate picture of the past can have important ramifications for the present. **Like the prior session, this session should be focused on reappraisal of the traumatic event(s)** *to the extent that there are remaining uncontextualized appraisals.* Psychoeducation about control can serve as a jumping-off point to determine how the couple's trauma appraisals disrupted or confirmed beliefs in this area.

In providing psychoeducation about control of oneself and others, the most important principles to convey are: that **(1) control applies to self and others; (2) stuck points involve the desire to over- and undercontrol self and others; and (3) healthy thoughts are balanced ones.** Orient the couple to *Getting U.N.S.T.U.C.K. Regarding Control (Handout 11.1)*.

*I'd like both of you to look at this handout about our next topic: control. When someone is traumatized, one's sense of the ability to exert control or influence over oneself and others can be disturbed. You'll notice that there are two columns on this handout: one focused on beliefs about self-control and one about control of others. Self-control is the belief that you have influence over your own decisions and behaviors, and other-control is the belief that you can control future outcomes in your relationships with others.*

*One of the things that can be most distressing about a traumatic event is that you have little to no control over the event. As a result, individuals with PTSD can have the stuck point that they must have control of themselves at all times or that they have no control any time. In other words, they have thoughts about over- or undercontrol. The same applies to beliefs related to partner and others. Individuals who were traumatized likely had others in control of them during or after the event. Individuals with PTSD can believe that others are seeking to unduly control them or that sharing control with another will result in their revictimization. They may go to the other extreme and give over their control to others because they don't expect to be able to share control.*

*Let's look at the questions related to self- and other-control to see whether you might have stuck points related to over- or undercontrol. . . .*

*The most important part of getting U.N.S.T.U.C.K. regarding control is to find and use balanced and realistic thoughts about control of self and other. Often, the desire to control is based on an interpretation of the traumatic event(s) that the situation was within your or others' control. The (erroneous) belief is that if enough control is exerted into the future, negative outcomes can be avoided. As we've discussed, accepting that there are situations, including the traumatic event, that are beyond one's maximal control efforts is very important to getting U.N.S.T.U.C.K. Undercontrol often comes from the appraisal that the traumatized individual had no control whatsoever during the traumatic event. The resulting belief is often that future traumatization is inevitable, and there is no expectation of control over those events.*

*In both cases, the thinking is extreme.*

*The resolution to stuck points about control is to use balanced, big-picture thoughts. Like trust, there are many things that one can attempt to exert control over, and there are varying degrees of control. There are everyday activities that we have varying degrees of control over, including what we wear (e.g., dressing up for work, wearing a uniform), what we eat, where we drive, and so on. There are also bigger ticket items for which we have varying levels of control, such as our children's behavior, health care decisions, partner's behavior, and so on.*

*Here are some examples of balanced, big-picture thoughts for healthy control [Getting U.N.S.T.U.C.K. Regarding Control (**Handout 11.1**)].*

## In-Session Practice: U.N.S.T.U.C.K. Regarding Control and Other Stuck Points

After the psychoeducation is complete, review with the couple their responses to the TIQ-I (*Handout 1.5*) as a starting point for identifying stuck points regarding control. This is also an opportunity to monitor progress of thoughts over the course of the therapy. The goal is to spend only a few minutes reviewing the TIQ-I so that they can identify their stuck points and begin their in-session U.N.S.T.U.C.K. process. The focus should be toward getting the couple to discuss these issues together, with you serving as a role model for Socratic dialogue.

*Let's look at what the two of you wrote at the beginning of therapy about your control beliefs. You have both done a lot of work since you first wrote these statements and so the thoughts you have now about control may already be different than the ones you wrote down weeks ago, but that's okay—we can note the changes, and reviewing your original responses will jump-start our discussion.*

After the couple shares their responses to the TIQ-I, have them turn their chairs to face each other to use the U.N.S.T.U.C.K. process to begin to address stuck points related to control and any other stuck points that have been prioritized to be addressed.

As in previous sessions, ask the partner to write the stuck point in the circle of *The Big Picture* (*Handout 11.2*) and coach the couple in their use of the U.N.S.T.U.C.K. process. It is important that you continue to strive to turn the work over to the couple so that they have as much experience as possible in using the U.N.S.T.U.C.K. process on their own. Continue to "plant" questions for the partner to ask to facilitate the Socratic dialogue between the couple.

After completing a worksheet, it is important to translate balanced thoughts into action. Consider with the couple whether there is any problem solving/decision making that they should embark upon. The problem solving can be as simple as "How can we carry out the 'K = Keep practicing' part of the U.N.S.T.U.C.K. process?"

While listening to the couple using the U.N.S.T.U.C.K. process, monitor for other stuck points that emerge during this session to be put on the *Stuck Point List* (*Handout 8.1*). The more stuck points that can be identified in session with the couple and placed on the list, the greater the chance that they can be effectively addressed out of session.

## Shrinking PTSD through Approach

From the *Avoidance List* (*Handout 3.2*), determine the next person, place, situation, or feeling that will be approached prior to the next session. Record the item on the *OOSA summary* (*Handout 11.3*) and ask the couple to write about how it went.

As in previous sessions, anticipate with the couple barriers to the success of carrying out the approach behavior and preemptively problem solve how those behaviors might be overcome. Refer them to the PROUD acronym in *Handout 4.3* to help strategize maximizing the benefits of the approach exercise.

## Out-of-Session Assignments

Orient the couple to the *OOSA summary* (*Handout 11.3*) for this session and point out the following assignments:

- Together, read the handout *Getting U.N.S.T.U.C.K. Regarding Control* (*Handout 11.1*).
- Have the couple use the U.N.S.T.U.C.K. process with *The Big Picture* (*Handout 11.2*) at least four times prior to the next session (more if they are willing). The PTSD+ partner should nominate at least one trauma-related cognition and the other partner should nominate any cognitions that he or she is struggling with (trauma related or not). Prioritize partners' stuck points that may impede their own (in dual-PTSD cases) or their partner's recovery (e.g., "My partner being distressed means her PTSD is worse"). Each partner should also nominate a relationship-related cognition that each has.

    By this point in the therapy, you are turning the therapy over to the couple, and part of their work outside of session is to be able to notice their own thoughts and then to apply the U.N.S.T.U.C.K. process to those noticed thoughts.

- Ask the couple to spend 5 minutes each day using their best communication skills with one another (*Handout 11.3*).
- Remind the couple of the item chosen from the *Avoidance List* (*Handout 3.2*) to be approached prior to the next session and ask them to record how it went.

## Check-Out

Ask the couple how the session was for each of them. Are there any lingering concerns or questions? What do they want to take with them from the session to improve their relationship and PTSD? Infuse hopefulness and predict success in completing the OOSAs as they leave the session.

HANDOUT 11.1

# Getting U.N.S.T.U.C.K. Regarding Control

**Beliefs Related to Self.** The belief that you have influence over your own decisions and behaviors.

*Individuals who have been traumatized experienced a lack of control in the situation, which can result in beliefs that they must retain control of themselves at all times in order to protect against future bad outcomes. Alternatively, they may believe that they have no control over the future.*

- Do you believe that you need to have control at all times?
- What would it mean if you were not in complete control in a situation?
- Do you believe that you have no control over events that happen to you?

**Beliefs Related to Partner and Others.** The belief that you can control future outcomes in interpersonal relationships.

*Individuals who have been traumatized often had others exert negative control over them during or after the event. As a result, they can believe that sharing control with another person will result in being a victim again, that other people are seeking to control them in negative ways, or that they will continue to give over their control to other people because they expect that they can't share control.*

- Do you believe that you must have control over others?
- Is it difficult to share control with others?
- Do you give up control to other people because you don't think it's possible to share control with others?

**There are many different types of things that can be controlled**—for example, what one wears, what and how much one eats and drinks, child outcomes, partner behavior.

**Control is on a continuum.** When people have been traumatized, they can get stuck by going to extremes in their thinking about control. Those extremes are to be overcontrolling or undercontrolling of themselves or others. Just like trust, control exists on a continuum and is dependent on the type of control.

### RESOLUTION: BALANCE

**Examples of more balanced, "big-picture" thinking are:**

- "I have control over many aspects of my life, but not all aspects.
- "Having control does not mean that a bad thing won't happen."
- "I have *influence* with my partner, but I don't want to control her choices."
- "Sharing control is part of a healthy relationship."

---

From *Cognitive-Behavioral Conjoint Therapy for PTSD: Harnessing the Healing Power of Relationships* by Candice M. Monson and Steffany J. Fredman. Copyright 2012 by The Guilford Press. Permission to photocopy this handout is granted to purchasers of this book for personal use only (see copyright page for details).

HANDOUT 11.2

# The Big Picture

**Noticed Thought:**

C: Feelings?

Behaviors?

K:

U = United and curious
N = Notice your thought
S = (Brain)Storm alternatives
T = Test them out
U = Use the most balanced
C = Changed feelings and behaviors
K = Keep practicing

From *Cognitive-Behavioral Conjoint Therapy for PTSD: Harnessing the Healing Power of Relationships* by Candice M. Monson and Steffany J. Fredman. Copyright 2012 by The Guilford Press. Permission to photocopy this handout is granted to purchasers of this book for personal use only (see copyright page for details).

HANDOUT 11.3

# Out-of-Session Assignments
## Session 11. Getting U.N.S.T.U.C.K. Regarding Control

1. Together, read *Getting U.N.S.T.U.C.K. Regarding Control* (*Handout 11.1*).

2. Use the U.N.S.T.U.C.K. process together at least four times prior to the next session. You should each work on two thoughts, one individually oriented and one relationship related, which can be drawn from the *Stuck Point List* (*Handout 8.1*). At least one of the individually oriented thoughts should be trauma related.

3. Spend 5 minutes each day using your best communication skills with one another. Place a checkmark below for each day you practiced.

| Sunday | Monday | Tuesday | Wednesday | Thursday | Friday | Saturday |
|--------|--------|---------|-----------|----------|--------|----------|
|        |        |         |           |          |        |          |

4. Shrinking PTSD through Approach:

_____

(people, place, situation, feeling)

Write about how it went:

_____

_____

**Next appointment:** _____ @ _____

---

From *Cognitive-Behavioral Conjoint Therapy for PTSD: Harnessing the Healing Power of Relationships* by Candice M. Monson and Steffany J. Fredman. Copyright 2012 by The Guilford Press. Permission to photocopy this handout is granted to purchasers of this book for personal use only (see copyright page for details).

# SESSION 12

# Emotional Closeness

---

### SUMMARY OF SESSION CONTENT

#### Goals

- Address overgeneralized here-and-now problematic core beliefs related to emotional closeness that may be maintaining PTSD and relationship discord.
- Emphasize that emotional closeness to self involves one's ability to soothe, tolerate, and manage one's own emotions and that healthy relationships include sharing and intimacy with close others.

#### Key Interventions

1. Review of Out-of-Session Assignments
   - *Getting U.N.S.T.U.C.K. Regarding Control* (Handout 11.1)
   - *The Big Picture* (Handout 11.2)
   - *Communication Skills Practice* (Handout 11.3)
   - *Shrinking PTSD through Approach* (Handout 11.3)

2. Introduction to Emotional Closeness (*Getting U.N.S.T.U.C.K. Regarding Emotional Closeness*, Handout 12.1)
   - Convey that traumatic events impact emotional closeness by seemingly confirming previously held negative beliefs or disrupting previously held positive beliefs.
   - Discuss the principles regarding emotional closeness as they apply to self and others (i.e., trauma and its consequences can disrupt people's sense of confidence in feeling their emotions and the experience of closeness with others).

3. In-Session Practice: U.N.S.T.U.C.K. Regarding Emotional Closeness and Other Stuck Points
   - Refer to the couple's TIQ-I (Handout 1.5) regarding barriers to emotional closeness.
   - Help the couple generate any stuck points related to emotional closeness.
   - Use problem solving/decision making after U.N.S.T.U.C.K.

4. Shrinking PTSD through Approach
   - Determine at least one place, situation, thing, or feeling to be approached.
   - Record the item on the *OOSA summary* (Handout 12.3).

5. Out-of-Session Assignments (Handout 12.3)
   - *Getting U.N.S.T.U.C.K. Regarding Emotional Closeness* (Handout 12.1)
   - *The Big Picture* (Handout 12.2)
   - *Communication Skills Practice* (Handout 12.3)
   - *Shrinking PTSD through Approach* (Handout 12.3)

6. Check-Out

*Administer the patient and partner versions of PCL/relationship happiness.

## Review of Out-of-Session Assignments

• *Getting U.N.S.T.U.C.K. Regarding Control* (Handout 11.1). Inquire whether either member of the couple had any questions about this handout.

• *The Big Picture* (Handout 11.2). Have the couple explain their use of the U.N.S.T.U.C.K. process on their respective cognitions. Reinforce the couple's hard work in doing the assignment, troubleshoot what got in the way of completing the assignment, and/or coach the couple on ways in which the U.N.S.T.U.C.K. procedure and use of *The Big Picture* could be optimized.

• *Communication Skills Practice* (Handout 11.3). Inquire about the couple's use of good communication skills since the last session.

• *Shrinking PTSD through Approach* (Handout 11.3). Review how the *in vivo* approach assignment went and reinforce any approach behavior and couple-level facilitation of such. Troubleshoot ways in which the couple may have accommodated avoidance. If the couple was successful in approaching an item off of the *Avoidance List* (Handout 3.2), in some way note this on their list (e.g., cross it out if no longer avoided, place a checkmark if previously assigned but still working on it).

## Introduction to Emotional Closeness

Transition out of the review of OOSAs to provide psychoeducation about **emotional closeness** as it relates to self and others. Like issues of trust, traumatic events often affect cognitions about emotional closeness, whether they confirm previously held negative beliefs or disrupt previously held positive beliefs. It is important to remember that accurate appraisal of the traumatic event(s) usually changes here-and-now thoughts about how close we can feel in relationship to oneself and others. Thus, a more accurate picture of the past can have important ramifications for the present. **Like the prior session, this session should be focused on reappraisal of the traumatic event(s)** *to the extent that there are remaining uncontextualized and processed appraisals.* Psychoeducation about emotional closeness can serve as a jumping-off point to determine how the couple's trauma appraisal disrupted or confirmed beliefs in this area.

In providing psychoeducation about emotional closeness, the most important principles to convey are that **(1) emotional closeness applies to self and others; (2) stuck points involve the fear of getting close to another person and the belief that your own emotions may be dangerous; and (3) healthy thoughts are balanced ones.** Orient the couple to *Getting U.N.S.T.U.C.K. Regarding Emotional Closeness* (Handout 12.1).

*It is probably no surprise to you that traumatic events can change the way you relate to other people and change the ease with which you experience and express your emotions. If you look at this handout on emotional closeness, you can see an outline of how emotional closeness is disturbed when someone is traumatized. You'll notice that there are two columns on this handout: one focused on beliefs you have about your own emotions and one focused on beliefs you have about being close to others. Emotional closeness with yourself may seem like a strange idea, but the way you relate to your own emotions and the beliefs you have about expressing them are very important for your well-being. Feeling emotionally confident means that you can experience, manage, and accept your emotions. Emotional closeness with others involves feeling close to another person through the sharing of your thoughts and feelings.*

*Traumatic events often involve other people, and the hurt and betrayal often included in that experience can make you afraid of connecting to others. It may seem safer to remain distant from them. Also, the strong emotions that these events caused may have made you fearful of the intensity of your emotions. As a result, individuals with PTSD can have the stuck point that it is unsafe to express feelings and that it is better to push them away. The same applies to beliefs related to your partner and others. Individuals who were traumatized usually have the belief that getting close to another person will only lead to hurt and more trauma. Individuals with PTSD often believe that sharing feelings with others will lead to pain and not to a satisfying feeling of connectedness.*

*Let's look at the questions related to self and other emotional closeness to see whether you might have stuck points in this area. The most important part of getting U.N.S.T.U.C.K. regarding emotional closeness is to find and use balanced and realistic thoughts about emotional closeness to self and other. Often, the fear of emotional closeness is based on an interpretation of the traumatic event(s) and also the assumption that all people, even your loved ones, are potentially threatening to you. The (erroneous) belief is that "If I get close to someone, I will get hurt."*

*You might also believe that avoiding your feelings or tamping down your sadness and anger will keep you safe and controlled.*

*In both cases, the thinking is extreme.*

*Here are some examples of balanced, big-picture thoughts for healthy emotional closeness:*

- *"Experiencing and showing my feelings is a sign of strength, not weakness."*
- *"Feelings cannot go on forever, unless I keep feeding them with my thoughts."*
- *"Feelings give me important information about myself and others."*

## In-Session Practice: U.N.S.T.U.C.K. Regarding Emotional Closeness and Other Stuck Points

After the psychoeducation is complete, review with the couple their responses to the TIQ-I (*Handout 1.5*) as a starting point for identifying stuck points regarding emotional closeness. This is an opportunity to monitor progress in their thoughts over the course of the therapy. The goal is to spend only a few minutes reviewing the TIQ-I so that they can identify their stuck points and begin their in-session U.N.S.T.U.C.K. process. The focus should be toward getting the couple to discuss these issues together, with you serving as a role model for Socratic dialogue.

After the couple shares their responses to the TIQ-I, have them turn their chairs to face each other to use the U.N.S.T.U.C.K. process to begin to address stuck points related to emotional closeness and any other stuck points that have been prioritized to be addressed.

Like in previous sessions, ask a partner to write the stuck point in the circle of *The Big Picture* (*Handout 12.2*) and coach the couple in their use of the U.N.S.T.U.C.K. process. It is important that you continue to strive to turn the work over to the couple so that they have as much experience as possible in using the U.N.S.T.U.C.K. process on their own. Continue to "plant" questions for the partner to ask to facilitate the Socratic dialogue between the couple.

After completing a worksheet, it is important to translate balanced thoughts into action. Consider with the couple whether there is any problem solving/decision making that they should embark upon. The problem solving can be as simple as "How can we carry out the "K = Keep practicing" part of the U.N.S.T.U.C.K. process?"

While listening to the couple using the U.N.S.T.U.C.K. process, monitor for other stuck points that emerge during this session to be put on the *Stuck Point List* (*Handout 8.1*). The more stuck points that can be identified in session with the couple and placed on the list, the greater the chance that they can be effectively addressed out of session.

## Shrinking PTSD through Approach

From the *Avoidance List* (*Handout 3.2*), determine the next person, place, situation, or feeling that will be approached prior to the next session. Record the item on the *OOSA summary* (*Handout 12.3*) and ask the couple to write about how it went.

As in previous sessions, anticipate with the couple barriers to the success of carrying out the approach behavior and preemptively problem solve how those behaviors might be overcome. Refer them to the PROUD acronym on *Handout 4.3* to help strategize maximizing the benefits of the approach exercise.

## Out-of-Session Assignments

Orient the couple to the *OOSA summary* (*Handout 12.3*) for this session and point out the following assignments:

- Together, read *Getting U.N.S.T.U.C.K. Regarding Emotional Closeness* (*Handout 12.1*).
- Have the couple use the U.N.S.T.U.C.K. process with *The Big Picture* (*Handout 12.2*) at least four times prior to the next session (more if they are willing). The PTSD+ partner should nominate at least one trauma-related cognition and the other partner should nominate any cognitions that he or she is struggling with (trauma related or not). Prioritize partners' stuck points that may impede their own (in dual-PTSD cases) or their partner's recovery (e.g., "My partner being distressed means her PTSD is worse"). Each partner should also nominate a relationship-related cognition that each has.

  By this point in the therapy, you are turning the therapy over to the couple, and part of their work outside of session is to be able to notice their own thoughts and then to apply the U.N.S.T.U.C.K. process to those noticed thoughts.

## Session 12. Emotional Closeness

- Ask the couple to spend 5 minutes each day using their best communication skills with one another (*Handout 12.3*).
- Remind the couple of the item chosen from the *Avoidance List* (*Handout 3.2*) to be approached prior to the next session and ask them to record how it went.

## Check-Out

Ask the couple how the session was for each of them. Are there any lingering concerns or questions? What do they want to take with them from the session to improve their relationship and PTSD? Infuse hopefulness and predict success in completing the OOSAs as they leave the session.

HANDOUT 12.1

# Getting U.N.S.T.U.C.K. Regarding Emotional Closeness

**Beliefs Related to Self.** These are beliefs about the value of your own emotions and, more specifically, your beliefs about how comfortable you are with being independent and reliant on yourself to experience, manage, and accept your emotions.

*Traumatic events are naturally associated with strong emotions that may have made you feel out of control of yourself and your emotions. This may have left you feeling that it is unsafe or out of control to feel your feelings. You may have also concluded that your feelings are bad and unsafe and that you are not able to accept or cope with them.*

- Do I believe that emotions are bad things to be stamped out, controlled, or at least not shown?
- Do I believe that I can soothe and calm myself when I am upset?
- How confident am I that I can handle difficult situations and the emotions that go with those situations?
- How confident am I that I can be emotionally hurt and recover from that again?

**Beliefs Related to Partner and Others.** The desire to connect and be close to others is one of our most basic human needs. Emotional closeness with others involves the feeling of being close to another person through sharing of your thoughts and, very importantly, your feelings.

*Traumatic experiences can confuse the desire to be close with others, including your closest loved ones, because most traumas involve other humans. The hurt and betrayal involved in trauma and/or the responses of other people after trauma can spread to your partner and other people in the world. You may have concluded that being close to someone will inevitably involve pain, betrayal, and more trauma.*

- Is sharing my feelings with my partner a good thing?
- Will sharing my thoughts and feelings *inevitably* lead to hurt?

## RESOLUTION: BALANCED THINKING

**Examples of more balanced, "big-picture" thinking are:**

- "Experiencing and showing my feelings is a sign of strength, not weakness."
- "Feelings cannot go on forever, unless I keep feeding them with my thoughts."
- "Feelings give me important information about myself and others."
- "When I shared my feelings before, I felt closer to my partner."
- "Not every single person in my life **has, or will,** betray me. If I am betrayed in some way, I can evaluate if and how I will be connected with that person into the future."

---

From *Cognitive-Behavioral Conjoint Therapy for PTSD: Harnessing the Healing Power of Relationships* by Candice M. Monson and Steffany J. Fredman. Copyright 2012 by The Guilford Press. Permission to photocopy this handout is granted to purchasers of this book for personal use only (see copyright page for details).

HANDOUT 12.2

# The Big Picture

Noticed Thought:

C: Feelings?

Behaviors?

K:

U = United and curious
N = Notice your thought
S = (Brain)Storm alternatives
T = Test them out
U = Use the most balanced
C = Changed feelings and behaviors
K = Keep practicing

From *Cognitive-Behavioral Conjoint Therapy for PTSD: Harnessing the Healing Power of Relationships* by Candice M. Monson and Steffany J. Fredman. Copyright 2012 by The Guilford Press. Permission to photocopy this handout is granted to purchasers of this book for personal use only (see copyright page for details).

HANDOUT 12.3

# Out-of-Session Assignments

## Session 12. Getting U.N.S.T.U.C.K. Regarding Emotional Closeness

1. Together, read *Getting U.N.S.T.U.C.K. Regarding Emotional Closeness* (Handout 12.1).

2. Use the U.N.S.T.U.C.K. process together at least four times prior to the next session. You should each work on two thoughts, one individually oriented and one relationship related, which can be drawn from the *Stuck Point List* (Handout 8.1). At least one of the individually oriented thoughts should be trauma related.

3. Spend 5 minutes each day using your best communication skills with one another. Place a checkmark below for each day you practiced.

| Sunday | Monday | Tuesday | Wednesday | Thursday | Friday | Saturday |
|--------|--------|---------|-----------|----------|--------|----------|
|        |        |         |           |          |        |          |

4. Shrinking PTSD through Approach: _____

   (people, place, situation, feeling)

Write about how it went:

_____

_____

**Next appointment:** _____ @ _____

---

From *Cognitive-Behavioral Conjoint Therapy for PTSD: Harnessing the Healing Power of Relationships* by Candice M. Monson and Steffany J. Fredman. Copyright 2012 by The Guilford Press. Permission to photocopy this handout is granted to purchasers of this book for personal use only (see copyright page for details).

# SESSION 13

# Physical Closeness

---

### SUMMARY OF SESSION CONTENT

#### Goals

- Encourage the couple to discuss how they use physical touch as a way of feeling close to one another and other people.
- Identify and address any stuck points that interfere with physical closeness.

#### Key Interventions

1. Review of Out-of-Session Assignments
   - *Getting U.N.S.T.U.C.K. Regarding Emotional Closeness* (Handout 12.1)
   - *The Big Picture* (Handout 12.2)
   - *Communication Skills Practice* (Handout 12.3)
   - *Shrinking PTSD through Approach* (Handout 12.3)
2. Introduction to Physical Closeness (*Getting U.N.S.T.U.C.K. Regarding Physical Closeness*, Handout 13.1)
   - Emphasize that physical closeness includes both sexual touching as well as physical affection that is nonsexual in nature.
   - Discuss the principles regarding physical closeness as they apply to self and others (i.e., trauma and its consequences can disrupt phases of the sexual response cycle as well as how people see themselves as sexual or sensual beings; physical closeness with others can be a way of increasing emotional closeness).
3. In-Session Practice: U.N.S.T.U.C.K. Regarding Physical Closeness and Other Stuck Points
   - Refer to the couple's TIQ-I (Handout 1.5) regarding barriers to physical closeness.
   - Help the couple generate stuck points related to physical closeness.
   - Use problem solving/decision making after U.N.S.T.U.C.K.
4. Shrinking PTSD through Approach
   - Determine at least one person, place, situation, or feeling to be approached.
   - Record the item on the *OOSA summary* (Handout 13.3).
5. Out-of-Session Assignments (Handout 13.3)
   - *Getting U.N.S.T.U.C.K. Regarding Physical Closeness* (Handout 13.1)
   - *The Big Picture* (Handout 13.2)
   - *Communication Skills Practice* (Handout 13.3)
   - *Shrinking PTSD through Approach* (Handout 13.3)
6. Check-Out

*Administer the patient and partner versions of PCL/relationship happiness.

## Review of Out-of-Session Assignments

- *Getting U.N.S.T.U.C.K. Regarding Emotional Closeness* (Handout 12.1). Inquire whether either member of the couple had any questions about this handout.
- *The Big Picture* (Handout 12.2). Have the couple explain their use of the U.N.S.T.U.C.K. process on their respective cognitions regarding emotional closeness. It is important that, as a therapist, you have truly handed the therapy process over to them because you are now three sessions away from completing the course of therapy. In this spirit, you become more of an observer of their shared process, coaching them on ways in which the U.N.S.T.U.C.K. procedure and use of *The Big Picture* was not optimized.
- *Communication Skills Practice* (Handout 12.3). Inquire about the couple's use of good communication skills since the last session.
- *Shrinking PTSD through Approach* (Handout 12.3). Review how the *in vivo* assignment went and reinforce any approach behavior and couple-level facilitation of such. Troubleshoot ways in which the couple may have accommodated avoidance. If the couple was successful in approaching an item off of the Avoidance List (Handout 3.2), in some way note this on their list (e.g., cross it out if no longer avoided, place a checkmark if previously assigned but still working on it). Identify and problem solve how to approach remaining big-ticket items that the couple is still avoiding.

## Introduction to Physical Closeness

The last session was spent helping couples understand how emotional intimacy may have been impeded by trauma-related beliefs and helping them to get "unstuck" from these beliefs in order to feel emotionally closer to one another. In this session, the focus is on helping couples understand how physical closeness may have been impeded by trauma-related beliefs and helping them to get unstuck from these beliefs in order to feel physically closer to one another.

The desire to connect and be close to others is one of our most basic human needs. Physical closeness involves the feeling of being close to another person through touch. Many people equate physical closeness with sexual intimacy. Emphasize to couples that *physical closeness includes both sexual touching as well as physical affection that is nonsexual in nature.*

In PTSD, both physical affection and sexual intimacy may have been affected by the traumatic experience(s) as a result of trauma-related beliefs about what it means to be touched by others. PTSD can also disrupt phases of the sexual response cycle. Orient the couple to *Getting U.N.S.T.U.C.K. Regarding Physical Closeness* (Handout 13.1).

*Traumatic experiences can confuse the desire to be physically intimate with others, including your closest loved ones. You may have concluded that others' intentions are negative (e.g., the only reason your partner wants physical contact with you is to gratify him- or herself sexually). You may feel uncomfortable being physically vulnerable and may have concluded that the way to stay safe and keep yourself from being hurt again is to avoid physical contact. Alternatively, you may believe that sex is the only way you can relate to another person.*

*PTSD can also cause changes in the way that people respond to one another sexually. For instance, if the trauma was interpersonal in nature and involved threat of bodily harm or a violation of one's physical boundaries (e.g., combat, sexual assault, mugging), physical contact with another person can be a trigger for reexperiencing and hyperarousal symptoms and make it hard to become and stay sexually aroused. The emotional numbing symptoms of PTSD can also lead to a decrease in sexual desire and arousal as well as a general aversion to feeling close to others physically.*

## In-Session Practice: U.N.S.T.U.C.K. Regarding Physical Closeness and Other Stuck Points

After the psychoeducation is complete, review with the couple their responses to the TIQ-I (*Handout 1.5*) as a starting point for identifying stuck points regarding physical closeness. This is an opportunity to monitor progress in their thoughts over the course of the therapy. The goal is to spend only a few minutes reviewing the TIQ-I so that the couple can identify their stuck points and begin their in-session U.N.S.T.U.C.K. process. The focus should be toward getting the couple to discuss these issues together, with you serving as a role model for Socratic dialogue.

*Let's look at what the two of you wrote at the beginning of therapy about your physical closeness beliefs. You have both done a lot of work since you first wrote these statements, and so the thoughts you have now about physical closeness may already be different from the ones you wrote down weeks ago, but that's okay—we can note the changes, and reviewing your original responses will jump-start our discussion.*

After the couple shares their responses to the TIQ-I, have them turn their chairs to face each other to use the U.N.S.T.U.C.K. process to begin to address stuck points related to physical closeness and any other stuck points that have been prioritized to be addressed.

Like in previous sessions, ask a partner to write the stuck point in the center of *The Big Picture* (*Handout 13.2*) and coach the couple in their use of the U.N.S.T.U.C.K. process. It is important that you continue to strive to turn the work over to the couple so that they have as much experience as possible in using the U.N.S.T.U.C.K. process on their own. Continue to "plant" questions for the partner to ask to facilitate the Socratic dialogue between the couple.

After completing a worksheet, it is important to translate balanced thoughts into action. Consider with the couple whether there is any problem solving/decision making that they should embark upon. The problem solving can be as simple as "How can we carry out the 'K = Keep practicing' part of the U.N.S.T.U.C.K. process?" For example, the couple could continue to make changes behaviorally by engaging in physically intimate, even if not sexually intimate, activities, such as holding hands, giving back rubs, and exchanging hugs.

While listening to the couple using the U.N.S.T.U.C.K. process, monitor for other stuck points that emerge during this session to be put on the *Stuck Point List* (*Handout 8.1*). The more stuck points that can be identified in session with the couple and placed on the list, the greater the chance that they can be effectively addressed out of session.

Some examples of stuck points related to physical closeness that we have encountered include:

- "It is unacceptable for me to relate to others through physical touch."
- "I'm damaged, and no one would want to be physically close to me."
- "(All) sex is unsafe and disrespectful."
- "Physical closeness will inevitably lead to my being hurt."
- "Sex is the only way I can relate to others."

After couple goes through the U.N.S.T.U.C.K. process, ask them to think about what changes they might like to put into place to enhance their physical closeness, defined as physical affection, sexual intimacy, or both.

## Shrinking PTSD through Approach

From the *Avoidance List* (*Handout 3.2*), determine the next person, place, situation, or feeling that will be approached prior to the next session. Record the item on the *OOSA summary* (*Handout 13.3*) and ask the couple to write about how it went.

As in previous sessions, anticipate with the couple barriers to the success of carrying out the approach behavior and preemptively problem solve how those behaviors might be overcome. Refer them to the PROUD acronym in *Handout 4.3* to help strategize maximizing the benefits of the approach exercise.

## Out-of-Session Assignments

Orient the couple to the *OOSA summary* (*Handout 13.3*) for this session and point out the following assignments:

- Together, read *Getting U.N.S.T.U.C.K. Regarding Physical Closeness* (*Handout 13.1*).
- Have the couple use the U.N.S.T.U.C.K. process with *The Big Picture* (*Handout 13.2*) at least four times prior to the next session (more if they are willing). The PTSD+ partner should nominate at least one trauma-related cognition and the other partner should nominate any cognitions that he or she is struggling with (trauma related or not). Prioritize partners' stuck points that may impede their own (in dual-PTSD cases) or their partner's recovery (e.g., "My partner being distressed means her PTSD is worse"). Each partner should also nominate a relationship-related cognition that each has.

    By this point in the therapy, you are turning the therapy over to the couple, and part of their work outside of session is to be able to notice their own thoughts and then to apply the U.N.S.T.U.C.K. process to those noticed thoughts.

- Ask the couple to spend 5 minutes each day using their best communication skills with one another (*Handout 13.3*).
- Remind the couple of the item chosen from the *Avoidance List* (*Handout 3.2*) to be approached prior to the next session and ask them to record how it went.

## Check-Out

Ask the couple how the session was for each of them. Are there any lingering concerns or questions? What do they want to take with them from the session to improve their relationship and PTSD? Infuse hopefulness and predict success in completing the OOSAs as they leave the session.

HANDOUT 13.1

# Getting U.N.S.T.U.C.K. Regarding Physical Closeness

**Beliefs Related to Self.** Beliefs about yourself as a sensual/sexual person reflect the extent to which you feel comfortable in your own skin and feel sexually attractive and experienced. They also relate to how acceptable you find it to derive pleasure through physical touch.

*Traumatic events are naturally associated with strong emotions that may have made you feel out of control of yourself and your emotions. They may have also left you feeling unsafe in your body. As a result, you may have concluded that being physically vulnerable puts you at risk of being hurt again.*

- Do I believe that it is acceptable for me to relate to others through physical touch?
- Do I believe that I'm damaged and that no one would want to be physically close to me?
- How confident am I that I can be in a situation that involves physical closeness and feel safe and respected?
- Will having physical closeness *inevitably* lead to hurt?

**Beliefs Related to Partner and Others.** The desire to connect and be close to others is one of our most basic human needs. Physical closeness involves the feeling of being close to another person through touch (e.g., physical affection and/or sexual touching).

*Traumatic experiences can confuse the desire to be physically intimate with others, including your closest loved ones. You may have concluded that others' intentions are negative (e.g., the only reason your partner wants physical contact with you is to gratify him- or herself sexually). You may feel uncomfortable being physically vulnerable and may have concluded that the way to stay safe and keep yourself from being hurt again is to avoid physical contact. Alternatively, you may believe that sex is the only way you can relate to another person.*

- Is having physical closeness with my partner a good thing?
- Is sex the only way I am able to relate to others?

### RESOLUTION: BALANCED THINKING

**Examples of more balanced, "big-picture" thinking are:**

- "Learning about what feels safe and pleasurable to me helps me feel more comfortable in my own body."
- "Sensuality and sexuality are a natural part of how we, as human beings, express ourselves."
- "Physical closeness with a safe, romantic partner is a sign of our closeness."
- "When I had physical contact before, I felt closer to my partner."
- "Sex is one of many ways to relate to another person through touch."

---

From *Cognitive-Behavioral Conjoint Therapy for PTSD: Harnessing the Healing Power of Relationships* by Candice M. Monson and Steffany J. Fredman. Copyright 2012 by The Guilford Press. Permission to photocopy this handout is granted to purchasers of this book for personal use only (see copyright page for details).

HANDOUT 13.2

# The Big Picture

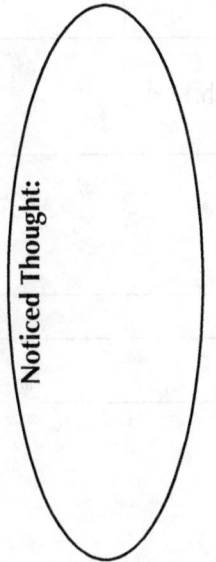

**Noticed Thought:**

C: *Feelings?*

Behaviors?

K:

U = United and curious
N = Notice your thought
S = (Brain)Storm alternatives
T = Test them out
U = Use the most balanced
C = Changed feelings and behaviors
K = Keep practicing

From *Cognitive-Behavioral Conjoint Therapy for PTSD: Harnessing the Healing Power of Relationships* by Candice M. Monson and Steffany J. Fredman. Copyright 2012 by The Guilford Press. Permission to photocopy this handout is granted to purchasers of this book for personal use only (see copyright page for details).

HANDOUT 13.3

# Out-of-Session Assignments
## Session 13. Getting U.N.S.T.U.C.K. Regarding Physical Closeness

1. Together, read *Getting U.N.S.T.U.C.K. Regarding Physical Closeness* (*Handout 13.1*).

2. Use the U.N.S.T.U.C.K. process together at least four times prior to the next session. You should each work on two thoughts, one individually oriented and one relationship related, which can be drawn from the *Stuck Point List* (*Handout 8.1*). At least one of the individually oriented thoughts should be trauma related.

3. Spend 5 minutes each day using your best communication skills with one another. Place a checkmark below for each day you practiced.

| Sunday | Monday | Tuesday | Wednesday | Thursday | Friday | Saturday |
|--------|--------|---------|-----------|----------|--------|----------|
|        |        |         |           |          |        |          |

4. Shrinking PTSD through Approach: _____

   (people, place, situation, feeling)

   Write about how it went:
   _____
   _____

**Next appointment:** _____ @ _____

---

From *Cognitive-Behavioral Conjoint Therapy for PTSD: Harnessing the Healing Power of Relationships* by Candice M. Monson and Steffany J. Fredman. Copyright 2012 by The Guilford Press. Permission to photocopy this handout is granted to purchasers of this book for personal use only (see copyright page for details).

# SESSION 14

# Posttraumatic Growth

## SUMMARY OF SESSION CONTENT

### Goals

- Encourage the couple to discuss how they have each grown individually or as a couple as a result of going through the trauma or treatment for PTSD.
- Identify and address any stuck points that interfere with posttraumatic growth.

### Key Interventions

1. Review of Out-of-Session Assignments
   - Getting U.N.S.T.U.C.K. Regarding Physical Closeness (Handout 13.1)
   - The Big Picture (Handout 13.2)
   - Communication Skills Practice (Handout 13.3)
   - Shrinking PTSD through Approach (Handout 13.3)

2. Introduction to Posttraumatic Growth (Getting U.N.S.T.U.C.K. Regarding Posttraumatic Growth, Handout 14.1)
   - Discuss the principles regarding posttraumatic growth as they apply to self and others (i.e., benefits or growth that occurred because of trauma or treatment, difficulties can coexist with positive consequences).

3. In-Session Practice: U.N.S.T.U.C.K. Regarding Posttraumatic Growth and Other Stuck Points
   - Help the couple generate any stuck points related to posttraumatic growth.
   - Use problem solving/decision making after U.N.S.T.U.C.K.

4. Shrinking PTSD through Approach
   - Determine at least one person, place, situation, or feeling to be approached.
   - Record the item on the *OOSA summary* (Handout 14.5).

5. Out-of-Session Assignments (Handout 14.5)
   - Getting U.N.S.T.U.C.K. Regarding Posttraumatic Growth (Handout 14.1)
   - The Big Picture (Handout 14.2)
   - Trauma Impact Questions–II (Handout 14.3)
   - What Have We Learned? (Handout 14.4)
   - Communication Skills Practice (Handout 14.5)
   - Shrinking PTSD through Approach (Handout 14.5)

6. Check-Out

**\*Administer the patient and partner versions of PCL/relationship happiness.**

## Review of Out-of-Session Assignments

- *Getting U.N.S.T.U.C.K. Regarding Physical Closeness* (Handout 13.1). Inquire whether either member of the couple had any questions about this handout.

- *The Big Picture* (Handout 13.2). Have the couple explain their use of the U.N.S.T.U.C.K. process on their respective cognitions regarding physical closeness. It is important that, as a therapist, you have handed the therapy process over to them, because you are now two sessions away from completing the course of therapy. In this spirit, you become more of an observer of their shared process, coaching them on ways in which the U.N.S.T.U.C.K. procedure and use of *The Big Picture* was not optimized.

- *Communication Skills Practice* (Handout 13.3). Inquire about their use of good communication skills since the last session.

- *Shrinking PTSD through Approach* (Handout 13.3). Review how the *in vivo* assignment went and reinforce any approach behavior and couple-level facilitation of such. Troubleshoot ways in which the couple may have accommodated avoidance. If the couple was successful in approaching an item off of the *Avoidance List* (Handout 3.2), in some way note this on their list (e.g., cross it out if no longer avoided, place a checkmark if previously assigned but still working on it).

## Introduction to Posttraumatic Growth

Introduce the idea that, despite the difficulties associated with having experienced a traumatic event(s) and the presence of PTSD in their relationship, the couple may still have noticed some positives that have come out of having experienced the event(s) or having PTSD in their lives and their relationship, including gains they experienced as a result of going through treatment together.

Note that some of these changes may have happened deliberately (e.g., partners now make a deliberate effort to spend more quality time together doing enjoyable things or made a decision to give back through volunteering), whereas others may have happened more implicitly (e.g., partners find themselves being more physically affectionate toward one another or sharing more with friends and family about their thoughts and feelings about various topics). Orient the couple to *Getting U.N.S.T.U.C.K. Regarding Posttraumatic Growth* (Handout 14.1).

*Most people, even those with PTSD, find that having experienced a traumatic event has brought about some unexpected positives. The presence of PTSD may also have also brought about unexpected benefits. In essence, some people have seen the value of making lemonade when given lemons. You may have been aware of some of these positives before participating in this treatment, or you may have come to see some while doing this work together. Some examples of benefits that people report are:*

- *"I realize how strong I am to have survived [the event]."*
- *"I was really brave to have done what I did."*
- *"I'm a 'survivor,' not a 'victim.'"*
- *"What doesn't kill me makes me stronger."*

- *"Talking about my trauma and PTSD has made me more open to exploring other things."*
- *"I can handle more than I thought"* or *"My partner can handle more than I thought."*
- *"As a result of having PTSD and going to treatment, I understand myself and my partner better."*
- *"I realize how committed my partner is to me."*
- *"My partner and I are closer as a result of going through this together."*
- *"I realize that although something bad happened to me in the past, my partner and I can decide together how to have the richest life possible going forward."*
- *"It has helped me/us develop our priorities."*

## In-Session Practice: U.N.S.T.U.C.K. Regarding Posttraumatic Growth and Other Stuck Points

After the psychoeducation is complete, ask the couple to turn their chairs toward each other to begin to address stuck points related to posttraumatic growth regarding the traumatic event or the presence of PTSD in their relationship, using *The Big Picture* (Handout 14.2). In determining the stuck point(s) to work on in this area, it is helpful to listen closely to the PTSD+ partner's reactions to the cognitive barriers to posttraumatic growth. When he or she hears about the different types of barriers, and as you solicit examples, the PTSD+ partner will often make comments about the specific barriers to his or her own posttraumatic growth. For instance, it is common for people to think that if they find something good out of this experience, it means that what they went through was not traumatic or that their negative feelings about the event are invalid.

*Many things can come from having experienced a traumatic event(s) and the PTSD symptoms related to it, some negative but also some positive. Although probably no one would wish to have experienced a traumatic event(s), some find, particularly at this stage of making sense of their experiences, that they may have grown as individuals and as a couple.*

*There are some thoughts that people have that can get in the way of being able to see positives that have come about as a result of the trauma(s). Some examples are:*

- *"If I see positives from having gone through the traumatic event(s), it means that what I went through wasn't traumatic."*
- *"If I see any good in the event, then it takes the perpetrator off the hook."*
- *"If I get better, it means that what I experienced wasn't so bad."*
- *"Once the person gets better, he or she may ask him- or herself, "Why did I suffer for so long?"—that is, why did the person wait so long to get treatment or why did earlier treatments not result in recovery from PTSD?*

*What, if any, thoughts do you have that have made or might make it hard to find some benefits of having gone through this experience?*

The use of Socratic dialogue can help couples develop balanced thinking about the fact that seeing positives does not mean that it was "okay" that the traumatic event happened, that it was not traumatic, or that their feelings about it are not justified. Rather, partners are aiming to hold both sides of the traumatic event constant at the same time (e.g., "As a result of having PTSD and then treatment, my partner and I understand each other better" or "Although something bad happened in the past, my partner and I can still have the richest life possible going forward").

After completing a worksheet, it is important to translate balanced thoughts into action. Consider with the couple whether there is any problem solving/decision making that they should embark upon. The problem solving can be as simple as "How can we carry out the 'K = Keep practicing' part of the U.N.S.T.U.C.K. process?" For example, "Remind myself that even though Katie and I are closer as a result of going through the recovery process from PTSD, it doesn't mean that what I went through wasn't traumatic."

## Shrinking PTSD through Approach

From the *Avoidance List* (*Handout 3.2*), determine the next person, place, situation, or feeling that will be approached prior to the next session. Record the item on the *OOSA summary* (*Handout 14.5*), and ask the couple to write about how it went.

As in previous sessions, anticipate with the couple barriers to the success of carrying out the approach behavior and preemptively problem solve how those behaviors might be overcome. Refer them to the PROUD acronym in *Handout 4.3* to help strategize maximizing the benefits of the approach exercise.

## Out-of-Session Assignments

Orient the couple to the *OOSA summary* (*Handout 14.5*) for this session and point out the following assignments:

- Together, read *Getting U.N.S.T.U.C.K. Regarding Posttraumatic Growth* (*Handout 14.1*).
- Have the couple use the U.N.S.T.U.C.K. process with *The Big Picture* (*Handout 14.2*) at least four times prior to the next session (more if they are willing). The PTSD+ partner should nominate at least one trauma-related cognition and the other partner should nominate any cognitions that he or she is struggling with (trauma related or not). Prioritize partners' stuck points that may impede their own (in dual-PTSD cases) or their partner's recovery (e.g., "My partner being distressed means her PTSD is worse"). Each partner should also nominate a relationship-related cognition that each has.

    By this point in the therapy, you are turning the therapy over to the couple, and part of their work outside of session is to be able to notice their own thoughts and then to apply the U.N.S.T.U.C.K. process to those noticed thoughts.

- Ask each partner to answer the questions included on the *Trauma Impact Questions–II* (*TIQ-II*; *Handout 14.3*). Reinforce that you want them to write about their beliefs as they

exist in the here and now, and not how they might have believed in the past, and to bring their responses with them to share in the next session.
- Complete *What Have We Learned?* (*Handout 14.4*) together in anticipation of the next and final session focused on reviewing their accomplishments and methods to prevent and manage lapses.
- Ask the couple to spend 5 minutes each day using their best communication skills with one another (*Handout 14.5*).
- Remind the couple of the item chosen from the *Avoidance List* (*Handout 3.2*) to be approached prior to the next session and ask them to record how it went.

## Check-Out

Ask the couple how the session was for each of them. Are there any lingering concerns or questions? What do they want to take with them from the session to improve their relationship and PTSD? Infuse hopefulness and predict success in completing the OOSAs as they leave the session.

HANDOUT 14.1

# Getting U.N.S.T.U.C.K. Regarding Posttraumatic Growth

**Beliefs Related to Self.** Although you did not wish for the traumatic event(s) to happen, some positives can come out of having experienced the event(s) or having PTSD in your life and your relationship. In essence, life has given you lemons, but you have made lemonade.

*Thus far, we have spent a great deal of time looking at how your thoughts have kept the PTSD going and talking about how changing your thoughts can change your emotions and behaviors. However, you may also have some concerns about what it means about you if you see positives associated with your traumatic experience(s).*

- If I see positives from the event, does it mean that what I went through was not traumatic?
- If I am better, does it mean that what I went through wasn't that bad?
- If it's possible to recover from PTSD, why did I suffer for so long?

**Beliefs Related to Partner and Others.** Although traumatic experiences and PTSD symptoms can negatively impact relationships, addressing them as a couple can actually strengthen relationships. An intimate relationship can be an important part of the healing process.

*During therapy, we've spent time looking at how changing your thoughts about other people, including your partner, has changed the way you feel about them and how you behave toward them. However, you may still have concerns about what it means about your relationships with other people if you think that you have grown or benefited in some way as a result of the trauma(s).*

- If I see any good in the event, does it take the perpetrator off the hook?
- If my partner sees that I have, in some way, benefited from the trauma, will he or she think that what I went through wasn't that bad?

## RESOLUTION: BALANCED THINKING

**Examples of more balanced, "big-picture" thinking are:**

- "I realize how strong I am to have survived [the event]."
- "Talking about my trauma and PTSD has made me more open to exploring other things."
- "I now know that I can handle really bad things happening to me."
- "As a result of having PTSD and then treatment, my partner and I understand each other better."
- "Although something bad happened, my partner and I can still have the richest life possible going forward."
- "Given what was known at the time, doctors and therapists did the best they could."

---

From *Cognitive-Behavioral Conjoint Therapy for PTSD: Harnessing the Healing Power of Relationships* by Candice M. Monson and Steffany J. Fredman. Copyright 2012 by The Guilford Press. Permission to photocopy this handout is granted to purchasers of this book for personal use only (see copyright page for details).

HANDOUT 14.2

# The Big Picture

**Noticed Thought:**

**C:** *Feelings?*

*Behaviors?*

**K:**

- **U =** United and curious
- **N =** Notice your thought
- **S =** (Brain)**S**torm alternatives
- **T =** Test them out
- **U =** Use the most balanced
- **C =** Changed feelings and behaviors
- **K =** Keep practicing

219

From *Cognitive-Behavioral Conjoint Therapy for PTSD: Harnessing the Healing Power of Relationships* by Candice M. Monson and Steffany J. Fredman. Copyright 2012 by The Guilford Press. Permission to photocopy this handout is granted to purchasers of this book for personal use only (see copyright page for details).

HANDOUT 14.3

# Trauma Impact Questions–II

Name: _____

1. What do I believe *now* about why the traumatic event(s) happened to me or my partner?

_____
_____
_____
_____
_____
_____
_____
_____
_____
_____
_____

2. What good things may have come about for us, individually and as a couple, as a result of my or my partner's having experienced the event(s)?

_____
_____
_____
_____
_____
_____
_____
_____
_____
_____
_____

*(cont.)*

---

From *Cognitive-Behavioral Conjoint Therapy for PTSD: Harnessing the Healing Power of Relationships* by Candice M. Monson and Steffany J. Fredman. Copyright 2012 by The Guilford Press. Permission to photocopy this handout is granted to purchasers of this book for personal use only (see copyright page for details).

# Trauma Impact Questions–II *(page 2 of 2)*

3. What do I believe *now* in the following areas, as each relates to *me, my partner, and others*?

    **Trust:**

    **Control:**

    **Emotional Closeness:**

    **Physical Closeness:**

HANDOUT 14.4

# What Have We Learned?

What specific ideas or skills have we learned through therapy that we want to remember and keep doing?

When we recognize that we are getting away from practicing these skills, we will:

---

From *Cognitive-Behavioral Conjoint Therapy for PTSD: Harnessing the Healing Power of Relationships* by Candice M. Monson and Steffany J. Fredman. Copyright 2012 by The Guilford Press. Permission to photocopy this handout is granted to purchasers of this book for personal use only (see copyright page for details).

HANDOUT 14.5

# Out-of-Session Assignments
## Session 14. Getting U.N.S.T.U.C.K. Regarding Posttraumatic Growth

1. Together, read *Getting U.N.S.T.U.C.K. Regarding Posttraumatic Growth* (Handout 14.1).
2. Use the U.N.S.T.U.C.K. process together at least four times prior to the next session. You should each work on two thoughts, one individually oriented and one relationship related, which can be drawn from the *Stuck Point List* (Handout 8.1). At least one of the individually oriented thoughts should be trauma related.
3. Each of you will complete the *TIQ–II* (Handout 14.3).
4. Together, complete *What Have We Learned?* (Handout 14.4).
5. Spend 5 minutes each day using your best communication skills with one another. Place a checkmark below for each day you practiced.

| Sunday | Monday | Tuesday | Wednesday | Thursday | Friday | Saturday |
|--------|--------|---------|-----------|----------|--------|----------|
|        |        |         |           |          |        |          |

6. Shrinking PTSD through Approach:

   _____
   (people, place, situation, feeling)

   Write about how it went:
   _____
   _____

   **Next appointment:** _____ @ _____

---

From *Cognitive-Behavioral Conjoint Therapy for PTSD: Harnessing the Healing Power of Relationships* by Candice M. Monson and Steffany J. Fredman. Copyright 2012 by The Guilford Press. Permission to photocopy this handout is granted to purchasers of this book for personal use only (see copyright page for details).

# SESSION 15

# Review and Reinforcement of Treatment Gains

---

**SUMMARY OF SESSION CONTENT**

### Goals

- Identify and reinforce the couple for the gains that they have made in therapy.
- Strategize with them how they will address challenges expected in the future.

### Key Interventions

1. Review of Out-of-Session Assignments
   - *Getting U.N.S.T.U.C.K. Regarding Posttraumatic Growth* (Handout 14.1)
   - *The Big Picture* (Handout 14.2)
   - *Trauma Impact Questions–II* (Handout 14.3)
   - *What Have We Learned?* (Handout 14.4)
   - *Communication Skills Practice* (Handout 14.5)
   - *Shrinking PTSD through Approach* (Handout 14.5)

2. Comparison of Pre- and Posttreatment *Trauma Impact Questions–II* (Handout 14.3)
   - Highlight changes that have occurred in the couple's thinking.
   - Predict further cognitive and behavioral changes with practice.

3. Review of *What Have We Learned?* (Handout 14.4) and Lapse Planning.
   - Review the couple's treatment goals from their *Treatment Contract* (Handout 1.3).
   - Review the major points of treatment and skills developed.
   - Encourage the couple to plan for future challenges and lapses.

4. Saying Good-Bye
   - Find a positive note on which to end the treatment.
   - Focus on the gains.
   - Consider a booster session for couples who are apprehensive about ending treatment.
   - Provide the couple with a certificate of completion.

---

\*Administer the patient and partner versions of PCL/relationship happiness.

## Review of Out-of-Session Assignments

- *Getting U.N.S.T.U.C.K. Regarding Posttraumatic Growth* (Handout 14.1). Inquire whether either member of the couple had any questions about this handout.

- *The Big Picture* (Handout 14.2). Have the couple explain their use of the U.N.S.T.U.C.K. process on their respective cognitions regarding posttraumatic growth.

- *Communication Skills Practice* (Handout 14.5). Inquire about the couple's use of the communication skills since the last session.
- *Shrinking PTSD through Approach* (Handout 14.5). Review how the *in vivo* assignment went and reinforce any approach behavior and couple-level facilitation of such. Troubleshoot ways in which the couple may have accommodated avoidance. If the couple was successful in approaching an item off of the *Avoidance List* (Handout 3.2), in some way note this on their list (e.g., cross it out if no longer avoided, check mark if previously assigned but still working on it).
- TIQ-I and -II and *What Have We Learned?* (Handout 14.4), as discussed next.

## Comparison of Pre- and Posttreatment TIQ

Bring the TIQ-I (*Handout 1.5*) written by each member of the couple to this session to allow for comparison with their TIQ-II (*Handout 14.3*) generated at the end of treatment. Have each member of the couple take turns reading their answers to the questions. The goal is to highlight changes that have occurred in their thinking. In addition, ask them to consider any remaining stuck points that may need to be further challenged and put these on their *Stuck Point List* (*Handout 8.1*). As an example, the posttreatment TIQ for Susan and Jake (Figure 15.1) shows the types of cognitive changes expected. Specifically, Susan's response to why the rape happened to her reflects greater acceptance of the event as it occurred at the time and appropriate reassignment of the blame from herself to the perpetrator. Susan also describes individual-level posttraumatic growth through her statement that she sees herself as stronger than she knew, and she and Jake both report couple-level posttraumatic growth through their responses that, as a result of going through the process of treatment together, they know each other better, appreciate one another more, and feel closer. Other cognitive changes are reflected in increased trust in one another, a greater ability to share control in their relationship, and more comfort being emotionally and physically intimate.

## Review of What Have We Learned? and Lapse Planning

*What Have We Learned?* (Handout 14.4) should be used as a starting point for discussing the couple's gains in therapy. The couple's treatment goals contained in their *Treatment Contract* (Handout 1.3) should be reviewed in this session to determine the extent to which they have been met. It is of utmost importance to give the couple positive feedback for finishing the treatment. Review major points of the treatment and skills developed, including:

- Understanding PTSD
  - Symptom clusters in PTSD
  - Dysregulation in the fight-or-flight system
  - Targets for intervention: behavioral strategies to address avoidance and emotional numbing and cognitive strategies to address problematic meaning making
  - Avoidance manifests in many forms (e.g., situations, people, places, feelings)

Name: SUSAN

1. **What do I believe *now* about why the traumatic event(s) happened to me or my partner?**

   I was simply at the wrong place at the wrong time. Just because I was drinking at a party doesn't mean that I deserved to be raped. It didn't cause the rape, though it may have made me less aware when it was happening. I didn't think the guy who did it was suspicious looking at the time. Now I think that not fighting back was probably the smartest thing I could have done, because he might have hurt me worse than he did.

2. **What good things may have come about for us, individually and as a couple, as a result of my or my partner's having experienced the event(s)?**

   Having gone through this therapy together, Jake understands me more. I also understand myself more. I see myself as stronger than I knew. Because I survived being raped, I realize that I am stronger than I thought. I also appreciate Jake more, because he has seen me through this.

3. **What do I believe now in the following areas, as each relates to *me, my partner, and others*?**

   **Trust:**

   I still struggle with trust, but I see myself trusting Jake much more. Going through this with him has strengthened my trust in him. I notice that I am not as wary of men, and I'm willing to take a few careful chances to test out my choices. Realizing that I made some good choices at the time of my rape has made me trust myself more.

   **Control:**

   I feel more in control of myself and my emotions. I don't feel like I need to control Jake as much. I realize that I influence people, but don't want to control them. They can influence me too, but I don't want to be controlled.

   **Emotional Closeness:**

   Jake and I are so much closer. My friendships are closer too, because I've opened up more about what has happened and what I've been doing to get better. It is not as scary to me to be around people who I don't know.

   **Physical Closeness:**

   Jake and I have made steps toward making our sex life better. At least I don't feel disgusted by sex at this point. I'm also willing to have other people hug me without wanting to vomit. And I'm more comfortable being around strangers and in social situations like parties.

   *(cont.)*

**FIGURE 15.1.** Susan's and Jake's Trauma Impact Questions–II.

Name: _Jake_

1. **What do I believe *now* about why the traumatic event(s) happened to me or my partner?**

   *I still believe that things just happen in life and we stand to learn from them. Susan has been able to change her beliefs about what happened, which has been great to watch.*

2. **What good things may have come about for us, individually and as a couple, as a result of my or my partner's having experienced the event(s)?**

   *Susan and I are closer because we have gone through this together. I feel like I know her much better— like she has come back from it. I also see what she and we are capable of when we put our hearts and minds to it.*

3. **What do I believe now in the following areas, as each relates to *me, my partner, and others*?**

   **Trust:**

   *I still trust myself and I trust Susan much more. She seems more predictable and stronger. Her trust in me seems to be growing. I don't trust others completely, but there are some people who are trustworthy.*

   **Control:**

   *I feel way more in control of myself in terms of our relationship. Susan is much less controlling of me because of talking about what happened to her in her rape and seeing how the past and the present are different. Others don't generally control me.*

   **Emotional Closeness:**

   *I feel like it is easier to be close to Susan. It also seems like Susan and I are more consistently close to each other. No other changes in my thoughts.*

   **Physical Closeness:**

   *It is really nice to feel like I have Susan back physically. Although we're not all the way there, I feel like she doesn't bristle every time I try to touch her. I like being physically affectionate with her and others whom I love.*

   **FIGURE 15.1.** *(cont.)*

- Importance of positivity
  - Noticing positive partner behavior
  - Approach exercises that double as shared rewarding activities
- Safety building
  - Recognizing early warning signs of own distress
  - Slowed breathing
  - Time-out as a strategy for containing conflict
- Communication
  - Listening/paraphrasing
  - Communication channels
  - Identifying, expressing, and reflecting feelings
  - Identifying and expressing thoughts
  - Problem solving/decision making
- Cognitive skills
  - U.N.S.T.U.C.K. process to address PTSD and relationship problems

It is important to stress to the couple that the communication and cognitive skills that they have developed will be further developed with **practice**. This therapy experience should be presented as a kick-start to a new *method* of communicating and approaching avoided issues. It will be a process that they can use into the future for meeting their individual and couple-oriented challenges. Predict that you expect further improvements based on their practice.

Encourage the couple to plan for future challenges and lapses. (We use "lapses" vs. "relapses" to indicate that the couple is never back to where they started and to convey that they may have future challenges or periods in which they are called upon to refine and/or use their developed skills.) The couple may be asked, "What will you do if 2 months from now you suddenly start experiencing conflict or more PTSD symptoms?" It is important to convey your confidence that they can meet increases in relationship conflict or PTSD symptoms, or other stressful events, with the skills acquired in treatment. These times should be seen as signals to use the skills they have acquired. Ask them which specific skills they would like to continue to practice.

## Saying Good-Bye

When saying good-bye to the couple, find a positive note upon which to end. This note may include their perseverance in completing the therapy, making some or many gains, and/or indicating that you enjoyed working with them. If there are sentiments that not as much was achieved as hoped, encourage them to consider that they will continue to make gains as they digest what has happened in the treatment and practice the skills. Focus on the gains that were made, irrespective of their size. For couples who exhibit significant apprehension about terminating, consider the possibility of a booster session 2 to 3 months after the last session as a goal toward which they can work while consolidating gains independent of you.

# References

Antony, M. M., & Roemer, L. (2011). *Behavior therapy.* Washington, DC: American Psychological Association.

Asmundson, G. J., Stapleton, J. A., & Taylor, S. (2004). Are avoidance and numbing distinct PTSD symptom clusters? *Journal of Traumatic Stress, 17,* 467–475.

Baker, A., Mystkowski, J., Culver, N., Yi, R., Mortazavi, A., & Craske, M. G. (2010). Does habituation matter? Emotional processing theory and exposure therapy for acrophobia. *Behavior Research and Therapy, 48,* 1139–1143.

Batten, S. V., Drapalski, A. L., Decker, M. L., DeViva, J. C., Morris, L. J., Mann, M. A., et al. (2009). Veteran interest in family involvement in PTSD treatment. *Psychological Services, 6,* 184–189.

Baucom, D. H., Shoham, V., Mueser, K. T., Daiuto, A. D., & Stickle, T. R. (1998). Empirically supported couple and family interventions for marital distress and adult mental health problems. *Journal of Consulting and Clinical Psychology, 66,* 53–88.

Baucom, D. H., Snyder, D. K., & Gordon, K. C. (2009). *Helping couples get past the affair: A clinician's guide.* New York: Guilford Press.

Baucom, D. H., Stanton, S., & Epstein, N. B. (2003). Anxiety disorders. In K. D. Snyder & M. A. Whisman (Eds.), *Treating difficult couples: Helping clients with coexisting mental and relationship disorders* (pp. 57–87). New York: Guilford Press.

Beck, A. T. (1976). *Cognitive therapy and the emotional disorders.* New York: International Universities Press.

Beck, A. T., Steer, R. A., & Brown, G. K. (1996). *Manual for the Beck Depression Inventory–II.* San Antonio, TX: Psychological Corporation.

Birrell, P. J., & Freyd, J. J. (2006). Betrayal trauma: Relational models of harm and healing. *Journal of Trauma Practice, 5,* 49–63.

Blake, D. D., Weathers, F. W., Nagy, L. M., Kaloupek, D. G., Gusman, F. D., Charney, D. S., et al. (1995). The development of a clinician-administered PTSD scale. *Journal of Traumatic Stress, 8,* 75–90.

Boeschen, L. E., Koss, M. P., Figueredo, A. J., & Coan, J. A. (2001). Experiential avoidance and posttraumatic stress disorder: A cognitive mediational model of rape recovery. *Journal of Aggression, Maltreatment and Trauma, 4,* 211–245.

Bouton, M. E. (2000). A learning theory perspective on lapse, relapse, and the maintenance of behavior change. *Health Psychology, 19*(1 Suppl.), 57–63.

Bouton, M. E. (2004). Context and behavioral processes in extinction. *Learning and Memory, 11,* 485–494.

Bradley, R., Greene, J., Russ, E., Dutra, L., & Westen, D. (2005). A multidimensional meta-analysis of psychotherapy for PTSD. *American Journal of Psychiatry, 162,* 214–227.

Brewin, C. R., Andrews, B., & Valentine, J. D. (2000). Meta-analysis of risk factors for posttraumatic stress disorder in trauma-exposed adults. *Journal of Consulting and Clinical Psychology, 68,* 748–766.

Bryant, R. A., & Harvey, A. G. (2002). Delayed-onset posttraumatic stress disorder: A prospective evaluation. *Australian and New Zealand Journal of Psychiatry, 36,* 205–209.

Buckley, T. C., Blanchard, E. B., & Hickling, E. J. (1996). A prospective examination of delayed onset PTSD secondary to motor vehicle accidents. *Journal of Abnormal Psychology, 105*, 617–625.

Byrne, C. A., & Riggs, D. S. (1996). The cycle of trauma: Relationship aggression in male Vietnam veterans with symptoms of posttraumatic stress disorder. *Violence and Victims, 11*, 213–225.

Carroll, E. M., Rueger, D. B., Foy, D. W., & Donahoe, C. P. (1985). Vietnam combat veterans with posttraumatic stress disorder: Analysis of marital and cohabitating adjustment. *Journal of Abnormal Psychology, 94*, 329–337.

Centers for Disease Control and Prevention, National Center for Injury Prevention and Control. (2011). *Understanding intimate partner violence.* Retrieved from www.cdc.gov/violenceprevention/pdf/IPV_factsheet-a.pdf.

Crane, D. R., Busby, D. M., & Larson, J. H. (1991). A factor analysis of the dyadic adjustment scale with distressed and nondistressed couples. *American Journal of Family Therapy, 19*, 60–66.

Craske, M. G., Kircanski, K., Zelikowsky, M., Mystkowski, J., Chowdhury, N., & Baker, A. (2008). Optimizing inhibitory learning during exposure therapy. *Behavior Research and Therapy, 46*, 5–27.

Davidson, J. R., Hughes, D., Blazer, D. G., & George, L. K. (1991). Post-traumatic stress disorder in the community: An epidemiological study. *Psychological Medicine, 21*, 713–721.

Dickstein, B. D., Vogt, D. S., Handa, S., & Litz, B. T. (2010). Targeting self-stigma in returning military personnel and veterans: A review of intervention strategies. *Military Psychology, 22*, 224–236.

Ehlers, A., Mayou, R. A., & Bryant, B. (1998). Psychological predictors of chronic posttraumatic stress disorder. *Journal of Abnormal Psychology, 107*, 508–519.

Epstein, N. B., & Baucom, D. H. (2002). *Enhanced cognitive-behavioral therapy for couples: A contextual approach.* Washington, DC: American Psychological Association.

First, M. G., Gibbon, M., Spitzer, R. L., & Williams, J. B. (1996). *Structured Clinical Interview for DSM-IV (SCID).* New York: Biometrics Research Department, New York State Psychiatric Institute.

Foa, E. B., Hembree, E. A., & Rothbaum, B. O. (2007). *Prolonged exposure therapy for PTSD: Emotional processing of traumatic events: Therapist guide.* New York: Oxford University Press.

Foa, E. B., Keane, T. M., & Friedman, M. J. (Eds.). (2009). *Effective treatments for PTSD: Practice guidelines from the International Society for Traumatic Stress Studies* (2nd ed.). New York: Guilford Press.

Fredman, S. J., Monson, C. M., & Adair, K. C. (2011). Implementing cognitive-behavioral conjoint therapy for PTSD with the newest generation of veterans and their partners. *Cognitive and Behavioral Practice, 18*, 120–130.

Frewen, P. A., & Lanius, R. A. (2006). Toward a psychobiology of posttraumatic self-dysregulation: Reexperiencing, hyperarousal, dissociation, and emotional numbing. In R. Yehuda (Ed.), *The psychobiology of post-traumatic stress disorder* (pp. 110–124). New York: Blackwell.

Freyd, J. J. (1996). *Betrayal trauma: The logic of forgetting childhood abuse.* Cambridge, MA: Harvard University Press.

Geiss, S. K., & O'Leary, K. D. (1981). Therapist ratings of frequency and severity of marital problems: Implications for research. *Journal of Marital and Family Therapy, 7*, 515–520.

Glenn, D. M., Beckham, J. C., Feldman, M. E., Kirby, A. C., Hertzberg, M. A., & Moore, S. D. (2002). Violence and hostility among families of Vietnam veterans with combat-related posttraumatic stress disorder. *Violence and Victims, 17*, 473–489.

Gold, J., Taft, C. T., Keehn, M., King, D. W., King, L. A., & Samper, R. (2007). PTSD symptom severity and family adjustment among female Vietnam veterans. *Military Psychology, 18*, 71–81.

Gottman, J. M., & Levenson, R. W. (1992). Marital processes predictive of later dissolution: Behavior, physiology, and health. *Journal of Personality and Social Psychology, 63*, 221–233.

Greenberg, P. E., Sisitsky, T., Kessler, R. C., Finkelstein, S. N., Berndt, E. R., Davidson, J. R. T., et al. (1999). The economic burden of anxiety disorders in the 1990s. *Journal of Clinical Psychiatry, 60*, 427–435.

Haney, C., Banks, C., & Zimbardo, P. (1973). Interpersonal dynamics in a simulated prison. *International Journal of Criminology and Penology, 1*, 69–97.

Hayes, S. C., & Gifford, E. V. (1997). The trouble with language: Experiential avoidance, rules, and the nature of verbal events. *Psychological Science, 8*, 170–173.

Hembree, E. A., Foa, E. B., Dorfan, N. M., Street, G. P., Kowalski, J., & Xin, T. (2003). Do patients drop out prematurely from exposure therapy for PTSD? *Journal of Traumatic Stress, 16*, 555–562.

Hoge, C. W., Castro, C. A., & Messer, S. C. (2004). Combat duty in Iraq and Afghanistan, mental health problems, and barriers to care. *New England Journal of Medicine, 350*, 13–22.

Institute of Medicine. (2007). *Treatment of posttraumatic stress disorder: An assessment of the evidence*. Washington, DC: National Academy of Sciences.

Jordan, B. K., Marmar, C. R., Fairbank, J. A., Schlenger, W. E., Kulka, R. A., Hough, R. L., et al. (1992). Problems in families of male Vietnam veterans with posttraumatic stress disorder. *Journal of Consulting and Clinical Psychology, 60*, 916–926.

Joseph, S. (1999). Social support and mental health following trauma. In W. Yule (Ed.), *Posttraumatic stress disorders: Concepts and therapy* (pp. 71–91). West Susses, UK: Wiley.

Kaniasty, K., & Norris, F. H. (2008). Longitudinal linkages between perceived social support and post-traumatic stress symptoms: Sequential roles of social causation and social selection. *Journal of Traumatic Stress, 21*, 274–281.

Kazantzis, N., Deane, F. P., & Ronan, K. R. (2000). Homework assignments in cognitive and behavioral therapy: A meta-analysis. *Clinical Psychology: Science and Practice, 7*, 189–202.

Kazantzis, N., Whittington, C., & Dattilio, F. (2010). Meta-analysis of homework effects in cognitive and behavioral therapy: A replication and extension. *Clinical Psychology: Science and Practice, 17*, 144–156.

Keane, T. M., Scott, W. O., Chavoya, G. A., Lamparski, D. M., & Fairbank, J. A. (1985). Social support in Vietnam veterans with posttraumatic stress disorder: A comparative analysis. *Journal of Consulting and Clinical Psychology, 53*, 95–102.

Kelly, K. A., Rizvi, S. L., Monson, C. M., & Resick, P. A. (2009). The impact of sudden gains in cognitive behavioral therapy for posttraumatic stress disorder. *Journal of Traumatic Stress, 22*, 287–293.

Kessler, R. C. (2000). Post-traumatic stress disorder: The burden to the individual and to society. *Journal of Clinical Psychiatry, 61*, 4–14.

Kessler, R. C., Sonnega, A., Bromet, E., Hughes, M., & Nelson, C. B. (1995). Posttraumatic stress disorder in the National Comorbidity Survey. *Archives of General Psychiatry, 52*, 1048–1060.

Kessler, R. C., Walters, E. E., & Forthofer, M. A. (1998). The social consequences of psychiatric disorders: III. Probability of marital stability. *American Journal of Psychiatry, 155*, 1092–1096.

King, D. W., Leskin, G. A., King, L. A., & Weathers, F. W. (1998). Confirmatory factor analysis of the clinician-administered PTSD scale: Evidence for the dimensionality of posttraumatic stress disorder. *Psychological Assessment, 10*, 90–96.

King, D. W., Taft, C. T., King, L. A., Hammond, C., & Stone, E. R. (2006). Directionality of the association between social support and posttraumatic stress disorder: A longitudinal investigation. *Journal of Applied Social Psychology, 36*, 2980–2992.

King, L. A., King, D. W., Fairbank, J. A., Keane, T. M., & Adams, G. A. (1998). Resilience-recovery factors in post-traumatic stress disorder among female and male Vietnam veterans: Hardiness, postwar social support, and additional stressful life events. *Journal of Personality and Social Psychology, 74*, 420–434.

Koenen, K. C., Stellman, J. M., Stellman, S. D., & Sommer, J. F. (2003). Risk factors for course of posttraumatic stress disorder among Vietnam veterans: A 14-year follow-up of American legionnaires. *Journal of Consulting and Clinical Psychology, 71*, 980–986.

Kubany, E. S., & Watson, S. B. (2002). Cognitive trauma therapy for formerly battered women with PTSD: Conceptual bases and treatment outlines. *Cognitive and Behavioral Practice, 9*, 111–127.

Linehan, M. (1993). *Cognitive-behavioral treatment of borderline personality disorder*. New York: Guilford Press.

McCann, I. L., & Pearlman, L. A. (1990). *Psychological trauma and the adult survivor: Theory, therapy, and transformation*. London: Brunner-Routledge.

Meis, L. A., Barry, R. A., Kehle, S. M., Erbes, C. R., & Polusny, M. A. (2010). Relationship adjustment, PTSD symptoms, and treatment utilization among coupled National Guard soldiers deployed to Iraq. *Journal of Family Psychology, 24*, 560–567.

Merikangas, K. R. (1982). Assortative mating for psychiatric disorders and psychological traits. *Archives of General Psychiatry, 39*, 1173–1180.

Milgram, S. (1974). *Obedience to authority: An experimental review.* New York: Harper & Row.

Milliken, C. S., Auchterlonie, J. L., & Hoge, C. W. (2007). Longitudinal assessment of mental health problems among active and reserve component soldiers returning from the Iraq War. *Journal of the American Medical Association, 298*, 2141–2148.

Monson, C. M., Fredman, S. J., & Adair, K. C. (2008). Cognitive-behavioral conjoint therapy for posttraumatic stress disorder: Application to Operation Enduring and Iraqi Freedom veterans. *Journal of Clinical Psychology: In-Session, 64*, 958–971.

Monson, C. M., Fredman, S. J., Adair, K. C., Stevens, S. P., Resick, P. A., Schnurr, P. P., et al. (2011). Cognitive-behavioral conjoint therapy for PTSD: Pilot results from a community sample. *Journal of Traumatic Stress, 24*, 97–101.

Monson, C. M., Fredman, S. J., & Dekel, R. (2010). Posttraumatic stress disorder in an interpersonal context. In J. G. Beck (Ed.), *Interpersonal processes in the anxiety disorders: Implications for understanding psychopathology and treatment* (pp. 179–208). Washington, DC: American Psychological Association.

Monson, C. M., Fredman, S. J., Dekel, R., & Macdonald, A. M. (in press). Family models of posttraumatic stress disorder. In J. G. Beck & D. M. Sloan (Eds.), *The Oxford handbook of traumatic stress disorders.* New York: Oxford University Press.

Monson, C. M., Gradus, J. L., Young-Xu, Y., Schnurr, P. P., Price, J. A., & Schumm, J. A. (2008). Change in posttraumatic stress disorder symptoms: Do clinicians and patients agree? *Psychological Assessment, 20*, 131–138.

Monson, C. M., Rodriguez, B. F., & Warner, R. (2005). Cognitive-behavioral therapy for PTSD in the real world: Do interpersonal relationships make a real difference? *Journal of Clinical Psychology, 61*, 751–761.

Monson, C. M., Schnurr, P. P., Resick, P. A., Friedman, M. J., Young-Xu, Y., & Stevens, S. P. (2006). Cognitive processing therapy for veterans with military-related posttraumatic stress disorder. *Journal of Consulting and Clinical Psychology, 74*, 898–907.

Monson, C. M., Schnurr, P. P., Stevens, S. P., & Guthrie, K. A. (2004). Cognitive-behavioral couple's treatment for posttraumatic stress disorder: Initial findings. *Journal of Traumatic Stress, 17*, 341–344.

Monson, C. M., Stevens, S. P., & Schnurr, P. P. (2005). Cognitive-behavioral couple's treatment for posttraumatic stress disorder. In T. A. Corales (Ed.), *Focus on posttraumatic stress disorder research* (pp. 251–280). Hauppauge, NY: Nova Science.

Morina, N., Stangier, U., & Risch, A. K. (2008). Experiential avoidance in civilian war survivors with current versus recovered posttraumatic stress disorder: A pilot study. *Behaviour Change, 25*, 15–22.

Mowrer, O. A. (1960). *Learning theory and behavior.* New York: Wiley.

Nezu, A. M., & Carnevale, G. J. (1987). Interpersonal problem solving and coping reactions of Vietnam veterans with posttraumatic stress disorder. *Journal of Abnormal Psychology, 96*, 155–157.

Norris, F. H., Friedman, M. J., & Watson, P. J. (2002). 60,000 disaster victims speak: Part II. Summary and implications of the disaster mental health research. *Psychiatry, 65*, 240–260.

Norris, F. H., Friedman, M. J., Watson, P. J., Byrne, C. M., Diaz, E., & Kaniasty, K. (2002). 60,000 disaster victims speak: Part I. An empirical review of the empirical literature, 1981–2001. *Psychiatry, 65*, 207–239.

North, C. S., Kawasaki, A., Spitznagel, E. L., & Hong, B. A. (2004). The course of PTSD, major depression, substance abuse, and somatization after a natural disaster. *Journal of Nervous and Mental Disease, 192*, 823–829.

Novaco, R. W., & Chemtob, C. M. (2002). Anger and combat-related posttraumatic stress disorder. *Journal of Traumatic Stress, 15*, 123–132.

O'Leary, K. D., & Williams, M. C. (2006). Agreement about acts of aggression in marriage. *Journal of Family Psychology, 20*, 656–662.

Ozer, E. J., Best, S. R., Lipsey, T. L., & Weiss, D. S. (2003). Predictors of posttraumatic stress disorder and symptoms in adults: A meta-analysis. *Psychological Bulletin, 129*, 52–73.

Pitman, R. K., Orr, S. P., Altman, B., Longpre, R. E., Poire, R. E., Macklin, M. L., et al. (1996). Emotional processing and outcome of imaginal flooding therapy in Vietnam veterans with chronic posttraumatic stress disorder. *Comprehensive Psychiatry, 37*, 409–418.

Price, J. L., Monson, C. M., Callahan, K., & Rodriguez, B. F. (2006). The role of emotional functioning in military-related PTSD and its treatment. *Journal of Anxiety Disorders, 20*, 661–674.

Resick, P., A., Monson, C. M., & Chard, K. M. (2008). *Cognitive processing therapy: Veteran/military version*. Washington, DC: Department of Veterans Affairs.

Resick, P. A., Williams, L. F., Suvak, M. K., Monson, C. M., & Gradus, J. L. (2012). Long-term outcomes of cognitive-behavioral treatments for posttraumatic stress disorder among female rape survivors. *Journal of Consulting and Clinical Psychology, 80*, 201–210.

Riggs, D. S., Byrne, C. A., Weathers, F. W., & Litz, B. T. (1998). The quality of the intimate relationships of male Vietnam veterans: Problems associated with posttraumatic stress disorder. *Journal of Traumatic Stress, 11*, 87–101.

Riggs, D. S., Rothbaum, B. O., & Foa, E. B. (1995). A prospective examination of symptoms of posttraumatic stress disorder in victims of nonsexual assault. *Journal of Interpersonal Violence, 10*, 201–214.

Rohrbaugh, M., Shoham, V., Spungen, C., & Steinglass, P. (1985). Family systems therapy in practice: A system couples therapy for problem drinking. In B. M. Bongar & L. E. Beutler (Eds.), *Comprehensive textbook of psychotherapy: Theory and practice* (pp. 228–253). New York: Oxford University Press.

Rothbaum, B. O., Foa, E. B., Riggs, D. S., & Murdock, T. (1992). A prospective examination of posttraumatic stress disorder in rape victims. *Journal of Traumatic Stress, 5*, 455–475.

Saunders, J. B., Aasland, O. G., Babor, T. F., & de la Fuente, J. R. (1993). Development of the Alcohol Use Disorders Identification Test (AUDIT): WHO collaborative project on early detection of persons with harmful alcohol consumption: II. *Addiction, 88*, 791–804.

Savarese, V. W., Suvak, M. K., King, L. A., & King, D. W. (2001). Relationships among alcohol use, hyperarousal, and marital abuse and violence in Vietnam veterans. *Journal of Traumatic Stress, 14*, 717–732.

Schumm, J. A., Fredman, S. J., Monson, C. M., & Chard, K. M. (2012). *Cognitive-behavioral conjoint therapy for PTSD: Initial findings for Operations Enduring and Iraqi Freedom male combat veterans and their partners*. Manuscript submitted for publication.

Sharpley, C. F., & & Cross, D. G. (1982). A psychometric evaluation of the Spanier Dyadic Adjustment Scale. *Journal of Marriage and the Family, 44*, 739–741.

Shaver, K. G., & Drown, D. (1986). On causality, responsibility, and self-blame: A theoretical note. *Journal of Personality and Social Psychology, 50*, 697–702.

Sheehan, D. V., Lecrubier, Y., Sheehan, K. H., Amorim, P., Janavs, J., Weiller, E., et al. (1998). The Mini-International Neuropsychiatric Interview (M.I.N.I.): The development and validation of a structured diagnostic psychiatric interview for DSM-IV and ICD-10. *Journal of Clinical Psychiatry, 59*(Suppl. 20), 22–33.

Sherman, M., Sautter, F., Jackson, H. M., Lyons, J. A., & Xiaotong, H. (2006). Domestic violence in veterans with posttraumatic stress disorder who seek couples therapy. *Journal of Marital and Family Therapy, 32*, 479–490.

Skinner, H. A. (1982). The drug abuse screening test. *Addictive Behaviors, 7*, 363–371.

Solomon, Z., Dekel, R., & Zerach, G. (2008). The relationship between posttraumatic stress symptom clusters and marital intimacy among war veterans. *Journal of Family Psychology, 22*, 659–666.

Spanier, G. B. (1976). Measuring dyadic adjustment: New scales for assessing the quality of marriage and similar dyads. *Journal of Marriage and the Family, 38*, 15–28.

Spielberger, R. L., & Lushene, R. E. (1989). *State–Trait Anxiety Scale*. Palo Alto, CA: Consulting Psychologists Press.

Straus, M. A., Hamby, S. L., Boney-McCoy, S., & Sugarman, D. B. (1996). The Revised Conflict Tactics Scale (CTS2): Development and preliminary psychometric data. *Journal of Family Studies, 17*, 283–316.

Taft, C. T., Monson, C. M., Schumm, J. A., Watkins, L., Panuzio, J., & Resick, P. A. (2009). Posttraumatic stress disorder symptoms, relationship adjustment, and relationship aggression in a sample of female flood victims. *Journal of Family Violence, 24*, 389–396.

Taft, C. T., Vogt, D. S., Marshall, A. D., Panuzio, J., & Niles, B. L. (2007). Aggression among combat veterans: Relationships with combat exposure and symptoms of posttraumatic stress disorder, dysphoria, and anxiety. *Journal of Traumatic Stress, 20*, 135–145.

Taft, C. T., Watkins, L. E., Stafford, J., Street, A., E., & Monson, C. M. (2011). Posttraumatic stress disorder and intimate relationship functioning: A meta-analysis. *Journal of Consulting and Clinical Psychology, 79*, 22–33.

Tarrier, N., Sommerfield, C., & Pilgrim, H. (1999). Relatives' expressed emotion (EE) and PTSD treatment outcome. *Psychological Medicine, 29*, 801–811.

Tee, J., & Kazantzis, N. (2011). Collaborative empiricism in cognitive therapy: A definition and theory for the relationship construct. *Clinical Psychology: Science and Practice, 18*, 47–61.

Van Ameringen, M., Mancini, C., Patterson, B., & Boyle, M. H. (2008). Post-traumatic stress disorder in Canada. *CNS Neuroscience and Therapeutics, 14*, 171–181.

van Minnen, A., Arntz, A., & Keijsers, G. P. J. (2002). Prolonged exposure in patients with chronic PTSD: Predictors of treatment outcome and dropout. *Behaviour Research and Therapy, 40*, 439–457.

Vasterling, J. J., & Brewin, C. R. (Eds.). (2005). *Neuropsychology of PTSD: Biological, cognitive, and clinical perspectives*. New York: Guilford Press.

Verbosky, S. J., & Ryan, D. A. (1988). Female partners of Vietnam veterans: Stress by proximity. *Issues in Mental Health Nursing, 9*, 95–104.

Veterans Health Administration, U.S. Department of Defense. (2004). *VA/DoD clinical practice guideline for the management of post-traumatic stress* (Version 1). Washington, DC: Author.

Weathers, F. W., Litz, B. T., Herman, J. A., Huska, J. A., & Keane, T. M. (1993, November). *The PTSD Checklist (PCL): Reliability, validity and diagnostic utility*. Paper presented at the 9th Annual Conference of the International Society for Traumatic Stress Studies, San Antonio, TX.

Whisman, M. A., Sheldon, C. T., & Goering, P. (2000). Psychiatric disorders and dissatisfaction with social relationships: Does type of relationship matter? *Journal of Abnormal Psychology, 109*, 803–808.

# Index

*f* following a page number indicates a figure; *t* following a page number indicates a table.

Acceptance session
   handouts for, 161–164
   introduction to acceptance, 153–156, 155*f*
   meaning making, 152–153
   out-of-session assignments, 152, 159–160
   overview, 151
   shrinking PTSD through approach, 159
   U.N.S.T.U.C.K. process and, 156–159, 159–160
Affairs. *see* Infidelity
Aggression
   blame (session 9), 169–170
   goal setting and, 61
   overview, 14
   personality disorders and, 38
   prevention strategies, 82–83
   relationship comorbidities and, 39–40
   relationship-level objective assessment and, 29–30
   safety building (session 2), 80–82
Alcohol use, 13, 35–36. *see also* Substance use
Ambivalence about the relationship, 40–41
Anger
   aggression and, 30
   cognitive-behavioral conjoint therapy (CBCT) for PTSD and, 4
   goal setting and, 61
   handouts regarding, 87, 94
   overview, 14
   prevention strategies, 82–85
Anxiety, 4, 29, 95
Appraisals, 14–15, 19–20, 180

Assessment
   case conceptualization and, 32–34
   determining appropriateness for CBCT for PTSD and, 26–27
   handouts regarding, 70–71
   individual-level objective assessment, 27–29
   multidyad groups and, 44–45
   ongoing assessment, 34
   overview, 27, 47–48
   relationship-level objective assessment, 29–32
   working with complex cases, 34–42
Avoidance
   handouts regarding, 67–69, 102, 103
   nonadherence to OOSAs and, 23–24
   psychoeducation regarding, 57, 58, 94–97, 95
   safety building (session 2), 80–83, 84
   shrinking PTSD through approach, 110–113
   substance use as, 35
   theoretical model for CBCT for PTSD and, 13, 15–16

**B**

Behaviors, 12–14, 80–83, 127–131, 130*f*–131*f*. *see also* Avoidance
Beliefs, 143, 180
Blame session
   handouts for, 176–178
   in-session practice, 172–174

235

Blame session *(cont.)*
 introduction to blame, 166–171
 out-of-session assignments, 166, 175
 overview, 165
 shrinking PTSD through approach, 174

## C

Case conceptualization, 32–34, 47–48. *see also* Assessment
Cognitive restructuring, 127–131, 130f–131f
Cognitive-behavioral conjoint therapy (CBCT) for PTSD
 alternative applications of, 42–46
 assumptions of, 20
 benefits of, 5–10
 coordinating with other interventions, 46–47
 implementation of, 21–24, 22f
 introduction to, 54–56
 mechanisms of PTSD and relationship problems and, 16–20, 17t
 overview, 3–5, 24–25, 47–48
 phases of, 54–56
 theoretical model for, 10–16, 12f
Communication channels, 106–107, 114, 118, 119, 120–121. *see also* Decision-making skills; Problem-solving skills; Sharing thoughts and feelings
Communication skills, 14, 17–18, 30–32, 97–98
Comorbidities, 4, 6, 29, 34–42
Complex cases, 34–42, 47–48
Conjoint therapy, 5–10, 56. *see also* Cognitive-behavioral conjoint therapy (CBCT) for PTSD
Control session
 handouts for, 194–196
 in-session practice, 191–192
 introduction to control, 190–191
 out-of-session assignments, 190, 192–193
 overview, 189
 shrinking PTSD through approach, 192

## D

Decision-making skills, 97–98, 114, 143–144, 146. *see also* Communication channels; Communication skills
Depression, 4, 29, 36–37, 69
Disclosure, 78–80, 153
Dissociation, 4, 6, 36. *see also* Emotional numbing system
Divorce, 8, 40–41
Dual-PTSD couples, 43–44, 79

## E

Emotional closeness session
 handouts for, 202–204
 in-session practice, 199–200
 introduction to emotional closeness, 198–199
 out-of-session assignments, 198, 200–201
 overview, 197
 shrinking PTSD through approach, 200
Emotional numbing system. *see also* Dissociation
 handouts regarding, 67–69
 overview, 13, 36
 psychoeducation regarding, 57, 58
 shrinking PTSD through approach, 197
Emotions, 15–16, 119. *see also* Feelings
Engagement in treatment, 7–10

## F

Fairytale thinking, 155, 171
Family functioning, 6–10. *see also* Relationship functioning
Feelings. *see also* Sharing thoughts and feelings
 avoidance and, 96
 communication channels, 106–109
 handouts regarding, 115
 in-session practice regarding, 109–110
 sharing thoughts and feelings - emphasis on feelings (session 4), 106–109
 shrinking PTSD through approach, 110–113
 U.N.S.T.U.C.K. process and, 127–131, 130f–131f
Forgiveness, 170–171

## G

Getting U.N.S.T.U.C.K. session. *see also* U.N.S.T.U.C.K. process
 handouts for, 134–137
 in-session practice, 132
 introducing the U.N.S.T.U.C.K. process, 127–131, 130f–131f
 out-of-session assignments, 127, 132–133
 overview, 126
 shrinking PTSD through approach, 132

## H

Happily-ever-after thinking, 155, 171
Hindsight bias, 14, 171

Homework. *see* Out-of-session assignments (OOSA)
Hopefulness, 27, 37, 140
Hyperarousal symptoms, 15, 30, 39, 56–58, 67–69
Hypervigilance, 14, 30

## I

Individual treatment, 6–7, 9, 45–46
Infidelity, 41–42, 81
Interpersonal factors in PTSD. *see* Relationship functioning
Intimacy, 110
Introduction to treatment session
  goal setting/treatment contract, 59–61, 60f
  handouts for, 63–71
  out-of-session assignments, 61–62
  overview, 53–56
  psychoeducation regarding PTSD, 56–59
  treatment overview, 54–56

## J

Just-world thinking, 154, 171

## L

Lapses
  overview, 35–36
  posttraumatic growth (session 14), 214, 217, 222, 224
  review and reinforcement of treatment gains (session 15), 225, 228
Listening and approaching session
  communication skills training, 97–98
  handouts for, 102–104
  in-session practice, 99–100
  listening skills, 98–100
  out-of-session assignments, 94, 100–101, 101f
  overview, 93
  psychoeducation, 94–97
Listening skills, 93, 97–100. *see also* Communication skills

## M

Meaning making of the trauma(s), 19–20, 151, 152–153

Memories, 9, 96, 153
Mental health symptoms, 26–27, 29, 34–42

## N

Nonadherence, 23–24, 37, 78
Numbing. *see* Emotional numbing system

## O

Out-of-session assignments (OOSA), 22, 22f, 23–24, 37, 42–43. *see also individual sessions*

## P

Pacing therapy sessions, 22, 22f
Paraphrasing skills, 97–98, 98–100. *see also* Communication skills
Personality disorders, 37–39
Physical aggression, 14, 38, 39–40, 81. *see also* Aggression
Physical closeness session
  handouts for, 210–212
  in-session practice, 205, 207–208
  introduction to physical closeness, 206–207
  out-of-session assignments, 205, 206, 208–209
  overview, 205
  shrinking PTSD through approach, 205, 208
Posttraumatic growth session
  handouts for, 218–223
  in-session practice, 213, 215–216
  introduction to posttraumatic growth, 214–215
  out-of-session assignments, 213, 214, 216–217
  overview, 213
  posttraumatic growth (session 14), 215–216
  shrinking PTSD through approach, 213, 216
Posttraumatic stress disorder (PTSD)
  assessment and, 27–29
  overview, 3–5, 56–59, 64, 67–69, 94–97
  relationship problems and, 16–20, 17t
Practice, 140, 141. *see also* Out-of-session assignments (OOSA)
Prevention strategies, 82–85, 88, 94
Problem solving to shrink PTSD session
  handouts for, 146–148
  in-session practice, 144
  introduction to problem solving/decision making, 143–144
  out-of-session assignments, 139–143, 145
  overview, 138

Problem-solving skills, 97–98, 114, 143–144, 146. *see also* Communication channels; Communication skills
Psychoeducation in general, 16–17. *see also individual sessions*
Psychosis, 26–27

# R

Recovery model of traumatic stress-related problems, 11–12, 12*f*
Reexperiencing cluster of symptoms, 56–57, 67–69
Relationship functioning. *see also* Family functioning
  ambivalence about being in the relationship, 40–41
  complex cases and, 39–42
  dual-PTSD couples and, 43–44
  emotional mechanisms and, 15–16
  engagement in treatment and, 7–10
  experiential avoidance and, 96–97
  handouts regarding, 67–69
  infidelity and, 41–42
  mechanisms of PTSD and relationship problems and, 16–20, 17*t*
  nonadherence to OOSAs and, 23–24
  nonromantic dyads and, 42–43
  psychoeducation regarding, 94–97
  relationship-level objective assessment and, 29–32
  safety building (session 2), 80–82
  theoretical model for CBCT for PTSD and, 12*f*
  therapeutic assumptions and, 20
R.E.S.U.M.E. Living acronym, 1, 16–20, 17*t*, 63
Review and reinforcement of treatment gains session
  comparison of pre-and posttreatment TIQ, 225, 226*f*–227*f*
  out-of-session assignments, 224–225
  overview, 224
  saying good-bye, 228

# S

Safety, aggression and, 39
Safety building session
  anger, 82–83
  negative behaviors as barriers to safety, 80–82
  overview, 73
  prevention strategies, 82–83
  review of out-of-session assignments, 74–78, 76*f*–77*f*
  time-out strategy, 83–85
  trauma focus and disclosure, 78–80
Self-report assessment, 26–27, 29–32. *see also* Assessment
Sexual aggression, 39–40, 81. *see also* Aggression
Sexual intimacy, 206–207. *see also* Physical closeness session
Sharing thoughts and feelings. *see also* Communication channels; Communication skills; Feelings; Thoughts
  communication skills training, 97–98
Sharing thoughts and feelings—emphasis on feelings session
  communication channels, 106–109
  handouts for, 114–117
  handouts regarding, 114, 117
  in-session practice, 109–110
  out-of-session assignments, 106, 113
  overview, 105, 108–109
  shrinking PTSD through approach, 110–113
Sharing thoughts and feelings—emphasis on thoughts session
  handouts for, 123–125
  identifying thoughts on the sharing channel, 120–121
  in-session practice, 121
  out-of-session assignments, 119–120, 122
  overview, 118
  shrinking PTSD through approach, 122
Shrinking PTSD through approach. *see individual sessions*
Situational factors, 155, 168–169, 169–170
Socratic dialogue, 153, 156–159, 191–192, 199, 216
Subjective Units of Distress Scale (SUDS) ratings, 18, 110
Substance dependence, 26–27, 35. *see also* Substance use
Substance use. *see also* Alcohol use
  aggression and, 39
  assessment and, 29
  avoidance and, 13
  determining appropriateness for CBCT for PTSD and, 26–27
  overview, 4, 35–36
Suicidality, 26–27, 36–37
Symptoms, 4, 11–16, 12*f*, 56–59, 64, 67–69
Symptom–system fit, 4, 35

# T

Terminating treatment, 19–20, 228. *see also* Review and reinforcement of treatment gains session

Theory, 10–16, 12*f*
Thinking patterns, 38, 127–131, 130*f*–131*f*
Thoughts, 96, 127–131, 130*f*–131*f*, 139, 140–143. *see also* Sharing thoughts and feelings
Time-outs, 83–85, 88, 94
Treatment contract
   handouts regarding, 65–66
   introduction to treatment (session 1), 53, 59–61, 60*f*
   review and reinforcement of treatment gains (session 15), 225, 228
Trust session
   handouts for, 185–188
   in-session practice, 182–183
   introduction to trust, 180–182
   out-of-session assignments, 180, 183–184
   overview, 179
   shrinking PTSD through approach, 183

## U

U.N.S.T.U.C.K. process, 18–19. *see also* Getting U.N.S.T.U.C.K. session; *individual sessions*

## V

Verbal aggression, 14, 38, 40, 81. *see also* Aggression
Violence, 29–30, 39–40. *see also* Aggression